The Mental Health and Wellbeing of Healthcare Practitioners

The Mental Health and Wellbeing of Healthcare Practitioners

Research and Practice

Edited by

Esther Murray

Barts and the London School of Medicine and Dentistry
Queen Mary University of London,
London, UK

Jo Brown

Barts and the London School of Medicine and Dentistry
Queen Mary University of London,
London, UK

WILEY Blackwell

Registered Office(s)
John Wiley & Sons, Inc., 111 River Street, Hoboken, NJ 07030, USA
John Wiley & Sons Ltd, The Atrium, Southern Gate, Chichester, West Sussex, PO19 8SQ, UK

Editorial Office
9600 Garsington Road, Oxford, OX4 2DQ, UK

For details of our global editorial offices, customer services, and more information about Wiley products visit us at www.wiley.com.

Wiley also publishes its books in a variety of electronic formats and by print-on-demand. Some content that appears in standard print versions of this book may not be available in other formats.

Library of Congress Cataloging-in-Publication Data
Names: Murray, Esther, editor. | Brown, Jo, 1957– editor.
Title: The mental health and wellbeing of healthcare practitioners :
   research and practice / edited by Esther Murray, Jo Brown.
Description: First edition. | Hoboken, NJ : Wiley, 2021. | Includes
   bibliographical references and index.
Identifiers: LCCN 2021007912 (print) | LCCN 2021007913 (ebook) |
   ISBN 9781119609513 (paperback) | ISBN 9781119609537 (adobe pdf) |
   ISBN 9781119609551 (epub)
Subjects: MESH: Burnout, Professional–prevention & control | Health
   Personnel–psychology | Compassion Fatigue–prevention & control
Classification: LCC R727.3 (print) | LCC R727.3 (ebook) | NLM WA 495 |
   DDC 610.69–dc23
LC record available at https://lccn.loc.gov/2021007912
LC ebook record available at https://lccn.loc.gov/2021007913

Cover Design: Wiley
Cover Image: © DrAfter123/Getty Images

Set in 10.5/13pt STIXTwoText by Straive, Pondicherry, India
Printed and bound by CPI Group (UK) Ltd, Croydon, CR0 4YY

C9781119609513_100621

Contents

Editor Biography

Prof Jo Brown EdD, MSc, BSc (Hons) Jo is Professor Emerita of Medical Education at Barts and The London School of Medicine and Dentistry, Queen Mary University of London. She was the former Deputy Vice Principal for Education at Queen Mary leading on Programme Review and the migration of education into a blended format in light of the COVID-19 pandemic. Her previous roles include being Head of Clinical Communication and Academic Director of the Student Experience at St George's, University of London. Jo has been teaching since 1992, has specialised in Clinical Communication as a topic since 1998 and her passion for the subject is infectious. In 2012 she won a prestigious National Teaching Fellowship award from Advance HE. She has a particular interest in providing academic support for students who struggle or fail whilst at university.

She is a curriculum leader and designer, an examiner and an external examiner and has spent two years visiting medical schools in The Netherlands and Canada to explore different conceptualisations of medical education. She is an experienced mentor of teachers in higher education and runs courses on teaching and learning as part of professional staff development. She developed and delivers postgraduate courses for senior doctors on the practical application of clinical communication in everyday clinical practice. She is a member of the Association for the Study of Medical Education and is a Principal Fellow of the Higher Education Academy. Her research interests center on the movement of learning from classroom to clinical environment and the challenges to learning in the clinical workplace.

Dr Esther Murray CPsychol AFBPsS SFHEA Esther has been a health psychologist for 13 years, initially working in cardiac care both in service improvement and psychological interventions for patients, later going on to a career in academia. Her early research was in chronic pain and its effect on doctor–patient communication. Esther has previous experience in psychological intervention in cardiac care and training NHS staff in communication skills.

Esther is the first researcher in the UK to explore the concept of moral injury in medicine, and was invited to present on the topic at the Institute of Pre-hospital Care Performance Psychology in Medicine Symposium in June 2017. Esther has been invited to present at national and international conferences for healthcare professionals, educators and students. Esther also delivers training on the moral injury and psychological wellbeing to London Ambulance Service's Advanced Paramedic Practitioners, the Counter Terrorism Specialist Firearms Officers of the Metropolitan Police and is a regular contributor to London HEMS Clinical Governance Days.

Esther has recorded podcasts for WEM, St Emlyns, The College of Paramedics and for the London Advanced Paramedics and East of England Ambulance Service, she also delivers wellbeing workshops at the Royal London Hospital for staff in theatres and at the Royal College of Emergency Medicine and the Intensive Care Society.

List of Contributors

Tony Allnatt
Royal London Hospital, London, UK
Barts Health NHS Trust, Whitechapel, London, UK

Ruth Anderson
Scottish Ambulance Service, Scotland, UK

Helen Bintley
Barts and The London School of Medicine and Dentistry, Queen Mary University of London, London, UK

Rebecca Connolly
Nottingham University Hospitals NHS Trust

Astrid Coxon
Institute of Psychiatry, Psychology & Neuroscience, King's College London, London, UK

Danë Goodsman
Barts and the London School of Medicine and Dentistry, Queen Mary University of London, London, UK

Bernice Hancox
Paramedic and Psychotherapist

Liz Harris
College of Paramedics, Bridgewater, UK

Andrea James
Brabners LLP Law Firm, Manchester, UK

Joanne Mildenhall
Faculty of Health & Applied Sciences, University of the West of England, Bristol, UK

Clare Morris
Barts and the London School of Medicine and Dentistry, Queen Mary University of London, London, UK
University of Cambridge, Cambridge, UK

Esther Murray
Barts and The London School of Medicine and Dentistry, Queen Mary University of London, London, UK

Rusty
St Emlyns, England, UK

Imogen Skene
Queen Mary University of London, London, UK

Gail Topping
Scottish Ambulance Service, Scotland, UK

Matthew Walton
National Health Service, London, UK

Jo Winning
Department of English, Theatre and Creative Writing, Birkbeck, University of London, London, UK

Tsz Lun Ernest Wong
Barts and the London School of Medicine and Dentistry, Queen Mary University of London, London, UK

Louise Younie
Barts and The London School of Medicine and Dentistry, Queen Mary University of London, London, UK

Introduction

Esther Murray

Barts and The London School of Medicine and Dentistry, Queen Mary University of London, London, UK

This book is the work of healthcare professionals and allied health professionals who have made the psychological wellbeing of their colleagues a part of their working lives. They are all, in one way or another, involved in the culture change which we know is needed in healthcare in order to keep staff safe and allow them to work in jobs that they love for as long as they want to. There are chapters written by psychologists, paramedics, general practitioners, anaesthetists and others; some are very personal stories of transformation, some are about interventions, some are traditional research and all focus on making spaces for those working in healthcare to be heard and find ways of managing the pressures of the job. Since starting work in a medical school it has become increasingly clear to me that there is a battle for the words to describe the experiences of staff as they deal with the trauma that they witness and also the day to day difficulties of understaffing, and the pressure to perform. There is certainly much more to say, and I see this book as the beginning, rather than the end, of the conversation.

I originally gave this book the title 'borrowed words' because I noticed how much words like resilience, burnout, compassion fatigue and so on were being used, all of which were developed in and borrowed from fields other than medicine. It has become increasingly common in medicine to borrow from other fields, probably the most well-known example is the borrowing of learning about human factors and safety from the field of aviation. Certainly this has been extremely useful in improving patient safety and developments in this area continue, always looking to develop more effective safety cultures in healthcare. (Chapter 13 of this book refers to such culture change.) Other borrowing is perhaps less useful, the wholesale dissemination of terms from other professional areas such as psychotherapy or social work will not apply in medicine and the uncritical adoption of these terms leads only to further resistance. The term resilience is an excellent example here. It originally describes the quality of materials to return to their original shape after being subjected to stressors such as bending or stretching, it was later applied in the field of child and developmental psychology in order to understand how children adapted to, and perhaps flourished despite, adversity. Its adoption in popular psychology has seen it applied in many different areas, perhaps without appropriate rigour. In healthcare it came to be seen as an entirely individual feature, and there was an emphasis on intervening to create more resilient staff. Such an endeavour was bound to fail given that not all members of staff would have started from the same baseline of stress and distress, or with the same individual traits, and that healthcare is not a system based on individuals but on teams. In fact, the research on resilience states that while there are individual traits which might be useful, they hinge largely upon the ability to enlist appropriate support when things are hard. So, while the ability to regulate one's emotions is an aspect of resilience, seeking a friend or colleague to talk to is an excellent way to regulate emotions. Failing to engage in sufficient depth with psychological concepts which might have been useful has meant that some concepts, such as resilience, have become buzzwords for management failure to properly support staff, seeming only to put the burden of coping back in the shoulders of staff rather than providing appropriate support and commitment to structural change.

It is true that what is needed is both structural change, team training *and* a focus on individual support and wellbeing. The chapters in this book focus on the ways in which staff experiences can be understood, in order to inform intervention; and the ways in which individuals have come together to create grassroots change.

PART 1

RESEARCH

CHAPTER 1

Borrowed Words in Emergency Medicine

How 'Moral Injury' Makes Space for Talking

Esther Murray

Barts and The London School of Medicine and Dentistry, Queen Mary University of London, London, UK

CONTEXT

In 2015 I started working at a medical school, it was an important move for me as I wanted to be a part of how doctors were trained, not only to ensure patients get the best possible care but also to understand how we can support doctors in practicing their profession without being harmed by it. I hadn't taken up a research post, but I had come along with a research idea, I wanted to know how it was that doctors (at this stage of my thinking) could practice for years, see terrible and upsetting things daily and not be affected by it. I had carried out some literature searches and found concepts like compassion fatigue and burnout, I had read reports of post-traumatic stress disorder in emergency responders, but what I had not seen was a systematic approach to understanding what was happening to doctors, and how we could combat it.

In my searches of 'doctor' and 'psychological' and 'trauma' I finally came across the writings of Jonathan Shay, a psychiatrist in the United States working with American war veterans in a VA hospital, this is a facility provided by the Veterans Health Association and serves veterans across the United States. His explanation of moral injury as one of the types of psychosocial harms that could be caused by repeated exposure to different types of traumatic events resonated powerfully with me. Although it did not seem to me that lots of doctors were suffering from diagnosable mental illness, it did seem that something was amiss. I could not really understand how it was that doctors were trained into, and then went on to practice their profession without the sort of regular supervision that psychologists are required to receive. I read about Balint groups, I heard about Schwartz rounds, but I could not find anything system-wide or systematic in the United Kingdom. What I did see was widespread discussions of burnout, equally widespread use of alcohol as a coping strategy, and a general sense that there was nothing to do but 'crack on'. This attitude that if you could not handle the pain then you should not be working in medicine at all was passed down to students and junior doctors.

Once I could pursue my area of interest at the medical school, I wanted to know if moral injury felt like a useful concept to doctors. I started my research with students in pre-hospital care, which is an area of medicine practiced by a variety of first responders such as doctors, nurses, paramedics, first aiders, remote medicine practitioners, voluntary aid workers, police, fire, and armed forces, it essentially covers any analytic, resuscitative, stabilising or preventative care given before the patient is admitted to hospital both at the scene of the incident and en route. The students I wanted to interview were all involved in either the Pre-hospital Care Programme (*PCP*) or the Intercalated Degree in Pre-hospital Medicine. The PCP is a student-led, staff supported programme in which students go out on shifts with the London Ambulance Service, mentored by specially trained paramedics. Students can join this programme from their second year at medical school. The intercalated degree (iBSc) in Pre-hospital Medicine is a year-long degree in the clinical, professional and psychosocial aspects of pre-hospital medicine for medical students. I was sure that pre-hospital care must be where the trouble lay since there was more evident trauma there than anywhere, with road traffic accidents, stabbings, shootings and suicide. The kind of medicine performed at the scene, the increasing likelihood of responding to terror attacks, and other kinds of mass casualties all seemed to suggest that pre-hospital care was where psychological trauma must occur. As time went on, it became clear that I was not quite right about what constitutes a 'traumatic event' for a doctor, and that doctors were only a small subsection of the people I should be thinking about, that no one was really thinking much about students and that no one had oversight of the situation or the degree of harm that had already been inflicted on healthcare professionals of all kinds.

Since I started out in 2015 the issue of the mental health of healthcare professionals has become more widely discussed. More and more work is being done at a national and local level to map the extent of the problem and there is recognition of the dearth of solid research that captures the experience of healthcare professionals, especially over time (General Medical Council (*GMC*), [1]). The terms usually used to describe the experience of being affected by healthcare work have often been borrowed from other areas of practice and it is worth tracing their various histories here.

Compassion Fatigue: Sinclair et al.'s [2] review of the use of the term compassion fatigue provides us with a useful frame for considering how we talk about the psychosocial effects of working in healthcare. Compassion fatigue refers to the gradual erosion of compassionate feelings towards, for example, patients, because of the high demands and stressful nature of the job. The point that Sinclair and colleagues are trying to make, though, is that the term 'compassion fatigue' like many similar terms in healthcare, is used without due care or appropriate rigour. Ledoux [3] points out that rather than trying to connote a lessening of compassion, as if compassion were a finite resource running in only one direction, it could be worth noting that much of the difficulty in maintaining compassionate attitudes is related to those things which thwart the expression of compassion such as long working hours, too few staff for too many patients, lack of rest for staff or opportunities to offload concerns. This conceptualisation is much closer to that of moral distress which has also been extensively explored in nurses and which is discussed below. Interesting observations can be made about those factors which might explain how they occur, it may be that some caring strategies are simply more prone than others to result in compassion fatigue, for example, a tendency to have a 'rescuing' style of caring will result in difficult feelings if the patient cannot be 'rescued'; a sense that perhaps the patient's illness is in part self-inflicted will interfere with compassionate feelings; difficult or disrupted patient interactions might mean that satisfaction cannot so easily be gained from the encounter and thus the good feelings which might offset the difficult or depleting feelings cannot necessarily be accessed.

An alternative conceptualisation of compassion fatigue is proposed by Charles Figley in his 1995 book 'Compassion Fatigue: Coping with Secondary Stress Disorder in Those Who Treat the Traumatised' in which compassion fatigue is a form of distress which arises from being exposed to the traumatic experiences of others'. The book focuses on the experiences of psychotherapists, trauma counsellors and others in the business of addressing the psychological needs of people who have undergone trauma. The term 'compassion fatigue' itself was borrowed from psychotherapists' experiences, as many of the terms used in understanding the emotional experiences of healthcare professionals have been borrowed. References to compassion fatigue as conceptualised by Figley, appear in papers about healthcare workers having been lifted wholesale and without further explanation in the text (see, for example, [4]). This is by no means a strange occurrence, in fact, in healthcare, the borrowing of learning from other industries is commonplace, with probably the most well-known example being the borrowing of safety and quality assurance techniques such as checklists, and learning on human factors from aviation. The learning from organisational psychology or other systems-based work, though, reminds us that it is not usually effective to take a concept wholesale from one area and apply it to another. It would be wiser to verify the appropriateness of the concept first. I have often wondered if the scientific background of much of medical practice has done it a disservice, in the end, meaning that concepts from social science do not look so credible as those from the physical sciences and are thus appropriated without much rigour, seeming 'good enough' or maybe 'harmless enough'.

Burnout: The concept of burnout was described by Christine Maslach in 1981 [5], as 'a psychological syndrome of emotional exhaustion, depersonalisation and reduced personal accomplishment' which can be the result of work demands which are principally relational in nature and where there is no opportunity to recharge. The term was developed to capture the experience of any person who worked 'in an intense involvement' with others, rather than those specifically in helping professions, this includes the criminal justice system and education. The result for workers is the sense that they are unable to do a good job, but also a disengagement from the people they had set out to serve, meaning that they are unable to access the potential good feelings which could be part of working with people. The concept is now very widely used in healthcare, a Google Scholar search in September 2020 of 'burnout healthcare professionals' returns 330 000 results.

Moral Distress: this concept was outlined by Jameton in 1984 in his book 'Nursing Practice: the ethical issues' [6] and refers to the effects of knowing what should be done for a patient, but being unable to do it because of situational and organisational constraints such as lack of time, staff or equipment. Most of the research in moral distress relates to nursing practice. The concept is of interest in this chapter since it highlights the relationship between organisational issues and personal, moral issues. This allows us to think of the healthcare professional's own agency in the workplace. Later work shows that to thrive at work, people need a sense of autonomy, belonging and competence and that this is as true for healthcare workers as for anyone else [7].

Secondary Trauma: refers to the stress experienced by helping those who have been traumatised. It is now listed in the Diagnostic and Statistical Manual of the American Psychiatric Association 5th Edition (DSM-5) as a potential aetiology for post-traumatic stress disorder (*PTSD*) (see below). This is an important development because it shows that there is a recognition of the powerful negative effects of helping work now. It would produce symptoms like hyperarousal, avoidance, intrusive thoughts and depression and anxiety type symptoms [8] and its effects have been explored in various professions, including healthcare.

Vicarious Trauma: describes the trauma that occurs from hearing the traumatic events that another has suffered, or in other ways being exposed to this trauma, including, one might assume, treating their physical injuries [8].

Note: The terms 'vicarious trauma' and 'secondary trauma' tend to be used exclusively from one another, sometimes the term secondary trauma is used to describe the after-effects of a primary trauma, for example, the loss of employment or relationship subsequent to primary trauma (such as domestic violence, violent crime, terrorism etc.).

Post-traumatic stress disorder (PTSD): this is a mental disorder that results from exposure to traumatic events that threaten the self or others [9]. The disorder is listed in the DSM-5 [10] and the symptoms include: intrusive memories and flashbacks, sleep disturbance, avoidance of places, people or things which remind the person of the event, possible dissociative symptoms, irritability, self-destructive behaviour and so forth. These symptoms need to have lasted for a month or more in order to meet diagnostic criteria. The inclusion, in the DSM-5, of PTSD caused by threats to others as well as self, recognises the effects of working as, for example, an emergency responder or in other areas where there is exposure to accidents and acts of violence, while not necessarily being the target of these acts of violence. The revised definition also recognises that one of the symptoms of PTSD will be persistent negative appraisals of the world, the self and the future [11].

Post-traumatic Growth: the idea that people can grow and develop as a result of adverse circumstances is not a new one and much has been written on the topic, especially by positive psychologists such as Maslow, Caplan and Csikszentmihalyi. Since the 1980s and 1990s much more research has been undertaken to explore this idea in a variety of areas such a bereavement, illness and accidents [12]. It describes profound transformative changes in relation to quite serious trauma, not just a resilience to these or maintenance of baseline wellbeing. It is an important consideration in a book about the mental health and wellbeing of healthcare practitioners given the likelihood of their exposure to traumatic events is so much greater.

Moral Injury: Moral injury, then, has been described in two ways, firstly, by Jonathan Shay as: the betrayal of what's right by someone who holds legitimate authority, in a high stakes situation [13] and as the result of: 'perpetrating, failing to prevent, bearing witness to or learning about acts that transgress deeply held moral beliefs or expectations' [14]. Shay's observations of veterans recovering from their experiences in the theatre of war highlighted the tenacious nature of the emotional reactions to these experiences. He spoke of their struggles to recover from the events which had rocked their view of themselves and of the world; even though they had undergone effective, evidence-based treatments for PTSD. Processing of events that he came to understand as morally injurious could only take place in peer groups where experiences among veterans were similar. Shay recognises his role as an outsider, conceptualising himself only as a facilitator of these discussions between people 'who know'.

The morally injurious event might take many forms, and indeed there is ongoing research to understand exactly what might constitute a morally injurious event (Journal of Traumatic Stress Special Issue June 2019), certainly the people I spoke to about my research had their own ideas about what was morally injurious for them. The resultant symptoms tend to follow a pattern, though, and this revolves mostly around shame and guilt, with their concomitant withdrawal from social networks. There are parallels with some of the aspects of guilt and disruption to world view which are now described in the latest iteration of the PTSD criterion and symptoms in the DSM-5 but in moral injury the source of this guilt and shame is different. Cognitive models of PTSD conceptualise the symptoms as the result of the interactions of the mind with extreme fear, that is, the world is appraised as an unsafe place in which terrible things can happen, the concept of moral injury suggests that the mechanism of action might be more closely related to feelings and thoughts about shame and guilt, that is, the world is a *wrong* place, in which terrible things are *allowed* to happen. The guilt and shame felt as a result of moral injury will not automatically extinguish over time if emotions are not effectively processed, researchers point out [15].

It may be that morally injurious events disrupt our individual worlds such that our attempts at meaning making fail and we are unable to resolve the cognitive dissonance we experience. Of course, assimilating events is part of our maturation as humans, but it seems that some events cannot be 'squared away' as easily as others.

Possibly the painful realisation of the wrongness of the world, and maybe ourselves in it, is extremely isolating. Certainly, feelings of guilt and shame tend to make us close off from our feelings, maybe by numbing them with food, drugs, alcohol or work, maybe by intellectualising our experience to the point where emotion is no longer present, but also by blaming others, by expressing anger (in lieu of sadness) all of these mean that we do not allow ourselves to access our individual experience of pain, sorrow and regret and thus do not move through it. As well as our individual experiences, we have our relationships with others which are also disrupted by moral injury.

In a special issue on Moral Injury in the Journal of Traumatic Stress, Litz and Kerig also point out that there are important cultural and individual factors to take into consideration with regard to understanding what might be morally injurious to any individual [16]. It is important to recognise a potentially bio-psycho-social-spiritual aspect to the practice of medicine, especially when healthcare practitioners work in teams, often in under-resourced settings and with little time or space to debrief, or benefit from peer support. Given the explosion of research into the psychosocial distress experienced by healthcare professionals and the urgent need to both explore and map the extent of the problem and to address the causes and consider the remedies, now may be the time to review and clarify the terms we might find useful to do that. In Canada, at the Canadian Institute for Public Safety Research and Treatment, the term 'Post-Traumatic Stress Injury' (www.cipsrt-icrtsp.ca) is preferred to PTSD because it recognises that the harms resulting from exposure to traumatic events may manifest as very significant symptoms but that these might not meet the diagnostic criteria for PTSD; equally to talk of injury rather than disorder calls to mind physical injuries, which can help remove some of the stigma which is often attached to mental health conditions. It is not unusual for workplace injuries to occur in medicine, and models like this one suggest that psychological or psychosocial injuries are as usual as needle sticks or injuries resulting from manual handling. Nor is it necessarily 'disordered' to experience strong and lasting psychological difficulty from traumatic situations.

Understanding the psychological harms of the workplace through a social psychological lens means that moral injury can be understood as happening to an individual but affecting the team, and the shared meanings in teams and work settings. It is important to remember that in many areas of medicine there is no long tradition of debriefing, or formal peer support whether after major incidents or even relatively routine incidents. Older physicians often talk to me about the erosion of safe spaces such as the doctors' mess, where cases could be discussed without fear of being overheard. Shift patterns have changed in many services now, resulting in long, 12-hour shifts with short handovers, there is increased lone working in pre-hospital care so that opportunities for peer support and rapid, informal, and timely debrief are eroded. There is no equivocation in the literature around these various topics; social support is extremely useful in mitigating the psychosocial impact of working in healthcare ([17], for example).

In Shay's initial understanding of moral injury, he discusses the role of leadership, how bad decisions by leaders left subordinates at risk. In any organisation, the actions of leaders and management affect the staff but as we have seen in the recent novel coronavirus pandemic, these actions can leave staff vulnerable to serious disease, disability and even death. This is probably as stark an example of the role of failures in leadership as that faced by Shay's Vietnam veterans. But even on a more average day, decisions at the highest level leave healthcare professionals vulnerable because of understaffing, inadequate hospital estates, insufficient equipment. The powerful hierarchies which exist in the National Health Service (*NHS*) and the services of allied health professionals often mean that staff have no recourse and feel that they cannot raise concerns in ways that will actually see them addressed. When leaders do not protect and defend the safety of their staff, they leave them emotionally and physically vulnerable. Since the NHS is an organisation which holds a particular place in the hearts of much of the nation, staff members find themselves in a constant position of dissonance. They are called on to provide a service for all but are insufficiently equipped to do so, which results in their being unable to offer a standard of care they can feel proud of and are constantly exhausted by demands they cannot meet. This means that their sense of self is under constant threat because 'who I am' and 'who we are' is not 'who we should be' but nor is it within their gift to change that.

DESCRIPTION

The initial research I undertook, alongside my colleagues Charlotte Krahe and Danë Goodsman explored the questions:

- Does the way in which medical students talk about their experiences in emergency medicine and pre-hospital care resonate with the concept of moral injury?
- If social support can be protective, to what degree do students feel they have access to this support and want to use it?

The study was envisaged as an exploratory study, and simply the first of a series across professional groups, exploring the lived experience of providing emergency medicine pre-hospital care, through the theoretical lens of moral injury. The focus group/interview schedule was adapted for healthcare populations from previous research on moral injury in military populations [18]. I conducted interviews and focus groups with students who were either on the intercalated degree in pre-hospital care, or involved in the pre-hospital care programme at the medical school, both of which would mean that they had exposure to traumatic incidents. The students knew me, as they had seen me attend symposia and so on in pre-hospital care. The students were offered the opportunity to amend transcripts but declined, nor did they take up the opportunity to review the findings. Questions were designed to be minimally distressing for students while exploring moral injurious experiences and symptoms resulting from moral injury, potential protective factors were also explored.

The data was analysed with thematic analysis (Braun and Clarke), through the theoretical lens of moral injury and there were themes which did indeed resonate with the concept of moral injury. Participants spoke of the ways in which the mechanism of injury affected how they felt about the job:

> 'it's always the ones with the violent connotations which are the hardest to process afterwards. . . when it's a violent attack there's an air about it of 'God, someone else has done this and it's up to us to reverse it'.

Sometimes a lack of resources caused problems:

> 'the paramedic had used up all his morphine. . . I felt so bad for this kid. . . he was in lots of pain and just basically lying on the floor and we couldn't do anything. I felt bad'.

In line with cognitive processing models, they found the clinical debrief to be useful, whether with a paramedic or physician who had also been on the scene:

> 'They know exactly what happened and you can say, well why did we decide to do this. . .then suddenly there is some kind of scientific underpinning, understanding that helps you process what's happened'.

Equally, they also talked about the need for emotional processing, 'Just sit down and understand and go, yeah, that's crap. . . talk me through it. Get everything out'. even when this was hard to do: 'You've got to make the effort, I find I have to make the effort. If I'm going to talk about it, I need to talk about it properly'.

Interestingly, this population did not talk about failures of leadership, or poor decisions made by leaders, but had unstinting admiration for their seniors and their extensive experience:

> 'he (the doctor) was like, okay, let's look for injury patterns because that's quite useful. I just remember thinking, oh my God. . . Obviously I was feeling a lot more than he was but that's just by virtue of him having – that's his job and that's his life'.

It was not until I started talking to other groups that I began to understand the issues that were arising with leadership, and also, that I had actually begun my exploration of moral injury in healthcare in the wrong place.

The research I undertook with students in pre-hospital care was meant to be the first step in a series of studies about whether moral injury was a concept that resonated with healthcare professionals. Once it was complete, I presented it with my collaborator, Charlotte Krahe, at a symposium in June 2017, two weeks after the fire at Grenfell Tower. I was overwhelmed by the response. I had thought there would be some interest in the topic, but I had not anticipated the number of people who would want to talk to me about their experiences, and their concern for themselves and their colleagues. It was this event that meant that I began to understand the extent of distress in paramedics and other ambulance staff, and in specialties such as intensive care, critical care, and, of course, emergency department staff.

Those who had not spoken to me at the time often wrote to me later, many were educators who wanted to know how to protect the students in their care:

> *'I actually think there is huge potential for use of the term "moral injury" to describe the feelings arising in clinicians and students from seeing patients in situ where there is severe deprivation, isolation, poverty, squalor, and sadness - a large part of what paramedics do and probably more frequently encountered than significant trauma, disturbing violence and serious illness.*
>
> *'The themes it (the published paper) has highlighted are the exact same that resonate across the entire student cohort and it's such a positive thing to see it professionally worked up. It points me in the right direction as to the best and better ways to keep our boys and girls as safe as possible'.*

Others sent me long emails about how moral injury resonated with their experiences, either because of the kinds of jobs they had seen, or the way they felt the system had treated them. At a conference, one physician told me: 'I just feel like a piece of meat on a conveyer belt. One day I'll fall off and they'll just put another piece of meat on'. It is clear that staff are feeling unsupported at work and we know from recent surveys that the degree to which staff will identify themselves as burnt out and stressed beyond their capacity to deal with it is worryingly high [1]. Since that first presentation of the research in June 2017, I have been invited to speak about moral injury at conferences, symposia and study days both in the United Kingdom and abroad. Clearly there is an appetite for discussion about moral injury and the psychosocial effects of working in healthcare more broadly.

FUTURE DIRECTIONS FOR RESEARCH AND INTERVENTION

There is no clear, recognised treatment for moral injury at the time of writing. There is speculation about the use of Acceptance and Commitment Therapy [19] given its focus on accepting the world as it is, with the good and the bad, and the equal emphasis on psychological flexibility. Treatments which focus on psychological flexibility are useful because they remind people that they are not their thoughts, that their thoughts occur independent of them and need not be engaged with, and if they are engaged with, their options for action and engagement can be of their own choosing. The ability to notice a world in which terrible things can happen and in which wonderful things also happen and not become fixated on either of these may be why this type of cognitive behavioural therapy would work.

There is a move among healthcare professionals to talk about preventing moral injury, which of course is not possible. The recent COVID pandemic has meant that the conditions for moral injury are all present – poor decisions made by leaders are causing death and post-viral disability, as well as economic devastation and healthcare workers are powerless to provide sufficiently 'good' care because they lack the resources to do so. While this experience is probably more pronounced in the United Kingdom and the United States, high death tolls among healthcare workers are common across the world which further adds to the sense of being put in harm's way. So, the moral injury is inevitable, and we need to plan for understanding how to support people through the grieving and meaning-making processes which might alleviate it.

Work is underway to develop questionnaires to understand moral injury in healthcare, with a view to mapping the problem and developing strategies to address it. Especially during the COVID-19 pandemic it has gained a great deal of traction and been mentioned in the popular press (Gerada, 16 October 2020) [20]. It has become clear that the incident which might be considered morally injurious differs greatly from one person to another. It is likely that the most effective interventions for managing harm will be those with which we are already familiar, that is, peer support, having time to talk, to debrief cases together, mapping both the clinical decisions and thinking about the feelings which these provoked. Healthcare professionals should be supported in finding solutions which work in their own settings and there will need to be a recognition of the structural issues that are affecting spaces for peer support.

REFERENCES

1. West, R. and Coia, D. (2019). Caring for doctors, caring for patients, General medical council. https://www.gmc-uk.org/-/media/documents/caring-for-doctors-caring-for-patients_pdf-80706341.pdf?la=en&hash=F80FFD44FE517E62DBB28C308400B9D133726450 (accessed 25 January 2020).

2. Sinclair, S., Raffin-Bouchal, S., Venturato, L. et al. (2017). Compassion fatigue: a meta-narrative review of the healthcare literature. *International Journal of Nursing Studies* 69: 9–24. https://www.sciencedirect.com/science/article/pii/S002074891730010X.

3. Ledoux, K. (2015). Understanding compassion fatigue: understanding compassion. *Journal of Advanced Nursing* 71 (9): 2041–2050. https://doi.org/10.1111/jan.12686.

4. Cocker, F. and Joss, N. (2016). Compassion fatigue among healthcare, emergency and community service workers: a systematic review. *International Journal of Environmental Research and Public Health* 13 (6): 618. https://www.ncbi.nlm.nih.gov/pmc/articles/PMC4924075.

5. Maslach, C. and Jackson, S.E. (1981). The measurement of experienced burnout. *Journal of Organizational Behavior* 2 (2): 99–113.

6. Jameton, A. (1984). *Nursing Practice: The Ethical Issues*. Englewood Cliffs, NJ: Prentice-Hall.

7. Kinman, G., Teoh, K., and Harriss, A. (2020). Supporting the well-being of healthcare workers during and after COVID-19. *Occupational medicine* 70 (5): 294–296. https://doi.org/10.1093/occmed/kqaa096.

8. Greinacher, A., Derezza-Greeven, C., Herzog, W., and Nikendei, C. (2019). Secondary traumatization in first responders: a systematic review. *European Journal of Psychotraumatology* 10 (1): 1562840.

9. CIPSRT (2020). www.cipsrt-icrtsp.ca. CIPSRT | Glossary of Terms. https://www.cipsrt-icrtsp.ca/en/resources/glossary-of-terms.

10. American Psychiatric Association (2013). *Diagnostic and Statistical Manual Of Mental Disorders: DSM-5*. American Psychiatric Association: Arlington, VA.

11. Miller, M.W., Wolf, E.J., and Keane, T.M. (2014). Posttraumatic stress disorder in DSM-5: new criteria and controversies. *Clinical Psychology: Science and Practice* 21 (3): 208–220.

12. Tedeschi, R.G. and Calhoun, L.G. (2004). TARGET ARTICLE: "Posttraumatic growth: conceptual foundations and empirical evidence". *Psychological Inquiry* 15 (1): 1–18.

13. Shay, J. (2014). Moral injury. *Psychoanalytic Psychology* 31 (2): 182–191.

14. Litz, B.T., Stein, N., Delaney, E. et al. (2009). Moral injury and moral repair in war veterans: a preliminary model and intervention strategy. *Clinical Psychology Review* 29 (8): 695–706.

15. Griffin, B.J., Purcell, N., Burkman, K. et al. (2019). Moral injury: an integrative review. *Journal of Traumatic Stress* 32 (3): 350–362.

16. Litz, B.T. and Kerig, P.K. (2019). Introduction to the special issue on moral injury: conceptual challenges, methodological issues, and clinical applications. *Journal of Traumatic Stress* 32 (3): 341–349.

17. Williams, R. and Kemp, V. (2020). Caring for healthcare practitioners. *BJPsych Advances* 26 (2): 116–128. https://doi.org/10.1192/bja.2019.66.

18. Currier, J.M., Holland, J.M., Drescher, K., and Foy, D. (2013). Initial psychometric evaluation of the moral injury questionnaire-military version. *Clinical Psychology & Psychotherapy* 22 (1): 54–63.

19. Nieuwsma, J., Walser, R., Farnsworth, J. et al. (2015). Possibilities within acceptance and commitment therapy for approaching moral injury. *Current Psychiatry Reviews* 11 (3): 193–206.

20. Alexander, M. (2021). The Guardian. https://www.theguardian.com/commentisfree/2021/apr/12/nhs-staff-moral-injury-distress-associated-with-war-zones-pandemic.

CHAPTER 2

What Does Creative Enquiry Have to Contribute to Flourishing in Medical Education?

Louise Younie

Barts and The London School of Medicine and Dentistry, Queen Mary University of London, London, UK

> *. . . to articulate subjective experience—if even privately, if only momentarily— constitutes a radical act that defies . . . depersonalization [1]*

CONTEXT

As a young GP new to the blood, sweat and tears of being alongside patients in the community, my image of the good doctor, knowledgeable about the body, its diseases and treatments, began to crumble. Patients attended with interwoven suffering of experience, emotions, trauma and disease, variously expressing themselves through body and mind. I was not prepared for the interpersonal work demanded from my consultations and at times, was lost in how I might transcend the chasm of meaning between my understanding and that of the patient. Seeking to engage future doctors with the complex interpersonal nature of practice, I began to explore Creative Enquiry, an approach which involves reflecting on lived experience through the arts. This work is counter-cultural, honouring practice, lived experience and subjectivity alongside the more traditional acquisition of facts and skills. Situating creative enquiry for flourishing in medical education requires consideration of the hidden curriculum, what creative enquiry might have to offer and what is meant by flourishing.

Medical education is a key transformative time in the life of our future clinicians, where they move from lay person to possessing the tools and skills of the doctor. The journey immerses students in a powerful cultural medium of competition, perfectionism and heroism [2]. These are features of the hidden curriculum, a concept described by Hafferty relating to what students *learn* through the medical school culture, structures and processes, rather than what they are *taught* as part of the formal curriculum [3]. The direction of travel tends towards negation of the human, intersubjective dimension, first for the patient and then for the doctor too. Proponents of patient or person-centred medicine call for greater attention to patients and their needs as human beings and collaborators in their own health, beyond that which a traditional biomedical approach to disease affords. At the other side of the 'patient–physician diad' [4], the doctor, trained as objective diagnostician can lose not just the personhood of the patient but also themselves in the process. Students describe being 'swallowed up' by medicine, losing their personal lives to their growing professional selves and 'the medical machine' [5].

Whilst the hidden curriculum potentially distances future doctors from their patients and their own humanity and suffering, creative enquiry can be a humanising force, connecting us with each other, ourselves and our emotions in meaningful ways [6, 7]. The arts connect through for example, slowing down perception, facilitating emotional expression, reframing experiences, inviting multiple perspectives and offering participatory and improvisational engagement with materials [8–11]. This chapter is a case study grounding some of these ideas within the context of medical education and showing what kinds of thinking and sharing are possible. I am not claiming that arts offer the only way of fostering connection (other examples include Schwartz rounds and Balint groups [12]), nor that it is easy to introduce arts for health and flourishing in the medical culture – there will be both resistance against creative enquiry approaches and a reckoning of the time and cost of facilitating such work [13].

Flourishing has been variously defined but in my work I draw on the concept of Eudaimonia, an Aristotolean concept relating not so much to pleasure and enjoyment (hedonia) although these make us happy in the short term, and more to authentic and meaningful engagement as well as personal growth [14–16]. Bringing the arts and flourishing together within medical education is a timely intervention. The rise in stress, burnout, anxiety and depression amongst medical students has raised concern [17, 18] and prompted both General Medical Council (*GMC*) and British Medical Association (*BMA*) further enquiry into the stressors that are negatively affecting students and doctors [19], carrying out surveys into doctor and student mental health [20]. On the arts front, there is a growing evidence base regarding arts for health in our patient populations documented in the recent All Party Parliamentary Group report [21], and in the largest evidence report to date, by the World Health Organisation [22]. The arts have been found to improve psychological and biological markers of stress as well as enhance wellbeing and mental health [23]. In the field of medical education, the literature evidences medical humanities penetrating the medical curriculum [11], however arts for health and flourishing of medical students rarely features.

DESCRIPTION

As a medical educator as well as a practicing GP my original focus when engaging students in creative enquiry, was around practice or practitioner development, seeking to expand the knowledges, processes and philosophies students have available to draw on in practice. These include personal as well as propositional ways of knowing, our subjective, intuitive and reflexive understandings alongside the facts and skills we can be tested on [24, 25]. However, I discovered that the creative enquiry process opened the door not just to practitioner development but also led to group and individual flourishing. One student captured this with a clay pot she formed with a small clay plant growing out of it as a metaphor for growth in the group. Before describing further what happened, two key approaches to creative enquiry innovations will be shared here.

Example 1   Creative Enquiry Introduction into Year 1 General Practice Attachment

Creative enquiry was introduced as an option in the year one GP attachment course I lead (2004–2010). This involved the whole year group of students having the *choice* to write a reflective essay *or* engage in creative enquiry in relation to a patient home visit [26, 27]. I supported medical student engagement with creative enquiry by explaining the concepts of right and left brain processing, engaging students in a drawing exercise and presenting former student creative work in the introductory lecture. Each year students stretched the creative space further pushing deeper into uncharted territory of visual art, video, dance, music compositions and more (www. outofourheads.net). After five years 85–90% students were choosing the creative enquiry option. What initially surprised me, more than the powerful aesthetics and well-crafted texts that the students began to produce, was the depth and breadth of thinking on practice and the introduction of the subjective and personal voice. Student work was evocative for the GP educators also, transforming perceptions of patients, of students and the value of the arts in medical education.

Example 2   Exploring the Creative Arts in Health and Illness

For the last 15 years I have been running and co-facilitating this practitioner development course, alongside arts for health consultants, therapists, patient artists and clinician artists, covering the fields of photography, clay work, creative writing, visual art, drama and music. It is an optional course which runs for an eight session or two-week block and has up to 13 students each time.

The different sessions often run to a similar structure where students:

- witness patient creative work (e.g. songs written by cancer patients),
- hear about the creative process (e.g. music therapy)

- create their own work (e.g. a co-created song)
- dialogue and reflect with their colleagues.

My introductory session involves considering how we listen to ourselves and how we listen to the other to introduce ideas around voice, ways of seeing, intersubjectivity and reflexivity. In another of the early sessions students are asked to bring in a meaningful object which helps to build group trust and sharing. The aim of these sessions is not so much to teach, as to educate, that is to draw out learning from students, to facilitate engagement with their lived experiences and ways of seeing, to encourage dialogue, exploration and multiple viewing points, helping them to become more aware of their own positioned nature.

A vulnerable leadership [28] approach is taken whereby the facilitator presences themselves as human in the room. Students are invited to articulate group rules – such as confidentiality and respect, and to consider their boundaries and how much they choose to share, given the potential for the creative process to open up inner doors to unexpected depths. Facilitators join in with the exercises to normalise the process and initial exercises are basic and grounding e.g. co-creative doodling, black pen on bits of paper and passing the papers around. This supports development of a 'freer . . ..relationship between gesture and sign' [29].

What I Learnt

Student Dialogue with Patients

Creative enquiry invites connection with the humanity of self and the other through more holistic engagement with the emotional and embodied dimensions of lived experience. In Example 1 above, where students engage in creative enquiry after a patient home visit, students comment on being 'more inclined to think of the patients as people with individual lives'. They describe how the arts help to 'consider the patient more deeply' because of, for example, having to 'think of how to display their issues visually' or spending time 'thinking about what colours represented the patient mood' or what image might communicate the narrative. After listening to a patient who suffered depression, one student describes choosing dark colours, painting a 'slumping figure' and using a Van Gogh painting style, who, as the student noted, suffered his own depression. The dark colours, wrote the student, also represents her own sadness and weariness after listening to the sufferings of this patient [26].

Students wrote about choosing the creative piece because of specifically wanting to 'capture his (the patient's) sadness. . .in a painting', or being more easily able to 'express emotions' and explore feelings:

The creative piece forced me to reflect on my own personal feelings and thoughts during the home visits: what story, idea imagery. . .impacted on me the most. . . and how could I convey that same intensity of feeling I had. . .to others [9].

This is illustrated in the following student text:

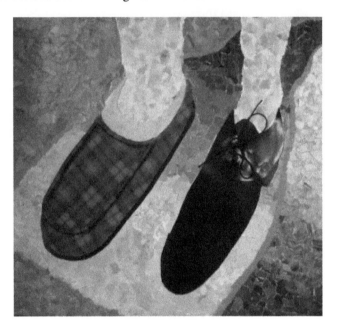

This student text called 'the slipper and the shoe' symbolises the patient's attitude towards life, to live and to never give up. First year medical student Sarah Saunders meets Charles (name changed) as he faces terminal cancer (the red on the path ahead). The dark behind him represents his difficult childhood and the light and yellow part the joy of his marriage. The blue part is the tears they both shed and connected through.

> . . . as Charles started to talk about his cancer, . . . the mood in the room changed. Almost without warning he began crying and I did not feel the sense of detachment that I had so hopefully thought I would. In the art work I have shown this part of the interview by a transition of blues running down the board. I have included this because I felt that it was an important moment for Charles and for me, as I think we both thought that we were strong enough, in very different ways, not to break down [9].

This is an example of how creative enquiry can explicitly engage students with what might often remain unexplored in the formal curriculum; the lived experience of being present to patients, witnessing suffering and how to manage the emotional boundaries. Research has found that intimate and emotionally laden encounters are a particular cause for feelings of professional uncertainty amongst students and junior doctors [30].

Student Dialogue with Each Other

In Example 2 detailed above, the creative arts course which engages a small group of self-selecting students with a number of creative enquiry workshops, their experience with the arts is similar. Students describe the value of engaging with the languages of the arts, connecting with emotions and with more personal ways of knowing. However, they also describe the challenges and vulnerability of making oneself more personally present, how they begin to learn with and from each other rather than engaging in a competitive manner, moving beyond seeking out the one right answer towards collaborative meaning-making. Creative enquiry facilitates a therapeutic space through the improvisational and process focussed learning environment, through the silence and creative exploration as well as the resulting quality of student connection and sharing. These dimensions will be explored below.

Sharing creations with colleagues and engaging with unfamiliar creative media can feel challenging. Even for those with leanings towards the arts, it may have been a long time since medical students engaged with creative writing, clay work or visual art. At the start of the course students are often tentative, generally not knowing each other particularly well. The fear of failure and exposure is written about in their reflective journals:

I am very apprehensive about writing something creative [8]

The painting that we did was not as terrifying as I thought it might be. . . I have not drawn or painted anything for years . . . [8]

One student pointed out how difficult it was to share her first creative text with the group because being creative demanded some kind of investment of the self. As time goes on it may be that personal engagement in creative expression is what enriches the group. Addressing the fear of creative expression, we encourage movement away from an outcomes focus of trying to produce technical masterpieces, towards improvisatory and exploratory ways of working with materials [31].

One thing which I found the most amazing about creative arts therapy is that there is no right or wrong way to do something [32].

Barbara Hepworth, one of our best known British Sculptors describes that while her right hand is at work the left hand listens as it grips the stone, for 'weaknesses, . . .flaws . . .or imminence of fractures' [33]. This kind of focussed listening and engagement, termed 'flow' [34] was experienced in the group, where 'each [was] consumed by what they were creating'.

One thing that really struck me about the process was how calming it was. There was no talking in the room for 20minutes because of how busy everyone was making their own art, and all you could hear was the rustling of materials or the gentle sound of pencil against paper. I felt like I was in a safe space [32].

As students feel safer, they progressively share more of themselves, elsewhere described as 'vulnerable reflection' [35]. A student image sketched other medical students as brightly coloured fish whilst she depicted herself as a small black fish at the bottom left hand corner of the painting. In their reflective journals other students wrote about their gratitude for her courage in sharing. Solidarity is built as they realise they are not alone.

> *I didn't expect to hear that other students felt out of their depth or like other people were more talented and bright than them so it was nice to discover I was not the only one. I didn't expect how open and honest everyone would be and it was refreshing [32].*

Through collective meaning-making and sharing, connections deepen. One participant described getting to know students better in this group over the last eight sessions, than he had other students over the last two years at medical school. Another student writes:

> *I remember writing lots that I felt privileged in the diary. . .because you don't usually get to see that side of people and I think it's a real honour when people decide that they feel comfortable enough or trust the group or you enough that they can open up like that [8].*

Student Dialogue with Themselves

One student who was well versed in visual art, had never before tried creative writing. After the creative writing session on the course, she began to use creative writing to process some of what she was going through and found it to be surprisingly powerful and helpful. She created an image to capture this, of an artist, face covered, painting her portrait. The Three Dimensional (*3D*) image of her face emerges from the page:

> *My painting is a self-portrait of me, writing. My hair is covering my face, this is to illustrate that when I initially pick up the pen, I am hiding from something; I am not in tune with myself. From the page I am writing on emerges my reflection; the idea that my identity is revealed to me as I write [27].*

This is a helpful illustration of how expression through the arts can facilitate or extend the dialogue we have with ourselves [36]. Other students also describe this experience:

> *The process [of writing a poem] requires you to be very honest and it stirred up many emotions that have remained dormant. . .It required me to be more honest with myself . . . . [8].*

> *. . .Poetic or artistic expression is a means by which innermost thoughts and feelings are given form so that they can be viewed and interpreted by their creators and by others. It has become evident how important it is to express these thoughts – to learn more about ourselves and to feel more at one in our own skin [8].*

It seems that through the creative process not only is vulnerable reflection with others possible, but a more vulnerable encounter with the self, and even the shadow sides of our experiencing which we might ordinarily seek to avoid [37]. Silence as well as creative expression may both be important facilitatory features in this work.

> *I found it helpful writing down what exactly I was finding difficult. It gave the challenges less power. . . [32].*

> *The periods of silence throughout the week are when I think I was able to sort out a lot of feelings and things I was experiencing in my personal life [32].*

Here one of the students makes the case for turning towards rather than away from what is difficult, the importance of which has also been described in creative enquiry work with junior doctors [38]. It is hard to argue against the importance of good eating, sleeping, exercising but perhaps there is also value in extending student engagement with their lived experiences and challenges through the arts or other kinds of group work.

> *In our lectures of wellbeing, we were often told that we need to make sure that we spend time with friends and pursue hobbies and interests outside of medicine. We were told to take regular breaks and to exercise. Though these suggestions are helpful, during this SSC I realised that all the wellbeing strategies we are taught teach us to allow Medicine to consume our whole lives, and to cope we should take intermittent short breaks to distract ourselves from the vacuum. I realised that true wellbeing, is facing what we are struggling with and not avoiding it, and finding the positives and solutions through that process [32].*

This deeply personal work of expression and exploration, using metaphor and symbol to extend reflection and understanding can be experienced as transformative [8].

> *To describe the Creative Arts Student Selected Components in two words would be: life changing. . . [32].*

> *. . .I believe that I learnt more about myself in the past two weeks than I have in my twenty-one years. I have been able to open up, when I have always kept my emotions and thoughts to myself. . . [32].*

FUTURE DIRECTIONS

What I have presented in this chapter is a snapshot into 15 years of creative enquiry work with medical students which shows that creative enquiry offers a learning environment of collaboration, enquiry and extended dialogue with the other and with ourselves. Through student quotes and creative work, I have sought to evidence ways in which creative enquiry can foster human flourishing alongside practitioner development work, actually two sides of the same coin – one relating to understanding the self and the vulnerability of human nature and the other to understanding of the humanity of others.

That this might lead to flourishing is endorsed by research by Satici et al. [39] into the connection between self-compassion (a concept which essentially relates to understanding our humanity) and flourishing amongst university students [39]. Students were asked to complete questionnaires that included the flourishing scale and the self-compassion scale. Analysis of responses found that self-kindness (rather than self-judgment), common humanity (versus isolation), and mindfulness (versus over identification) were positively related to flourishing [39]. *Self-kindness* means being warm and understanding towards oneself in our inadequacies and failings rather than ignoring pain, or being self-critical. *Common humanity* refers to understanding that we all fall short, make mistakes, feel inadequate and this can be a point of connection rather than isolation. *Mindfulness* is described as engaging with negative emotions in a balanced way, not suppressing or exaggerating them [39]. Creative enquiry offers an environment that invites kindness and connection in vulnerability as well the arts themselves offering other languages to gently explore emotions that might be difficult to articulate.

Lee Roze des Ordons et al. [40] explore humanity in relation to both patient care and physician wellness (similar to my concepts of practitioner development and human flourishing, respectively) through semi-structured interviews with faculty. Five themes relating to shared humanity emerged. These all find resonance in my description of creative enquiry above. They are *Whole person care* – engaging with psycho-socio-emotional dimensions of personhood, *Valuing* – respect for a person's intrinsic value, *Perspective taking* – engaging with other perspectives and suspending judgment regarding other worldviews, *Recognising universality* – the shared elements of the human condition beyond professional boundaries and finally *Relational focus* – becoming part of another's story and reciprocally being transformed and changed through entering another's world. The authors mention the need for 'creative imagining' on how to embed this work in the undergraduate curriculum. What I have offered are examples of ways in which this kind of humanism is already being invited.

However, as intimated in my introduction, creative enquiry in medical education is not without its risks and application of these creative enquiry examples to medical education in general also has its limitations. Key risks in this kind of work include the risk of student exposure or difficulty in maintaining their boundaries. Careful facilitation is necessary with vulnerable leadership creating a space where our humanity and frailty are accepted and welcomed as well as respecting student privacy and holding back. For arts therapists and arts for health practitioners making space for the student voice may come more naturally than clinician educators for whom space and silence can be deeply counter-cultural [41]. 'Artist of the invisible' is a term given to the art of facilitating a transformative learning group [42]. It is a helpful concept which can be applied to creative enquiry group facilitation to explain the creativity needed in order to craft a conducive group environment.

Emotional engagement can be draining and usually in each course at some point tears are shed. Research on the small group work described above found evidence of students questioning the emotional expression within the group, for example proposing more warning prior to emotional sessions e.g. where an artist/painter told his life story regarding his diagnosis and recurrence of lymphoma [8]. The group has always worked well, however, to hold a safe space and many comment on the heavier emotional sessions being the most beneficial, though not always enjoying them [8]. Also, life as a doctor is inevitably one which involves the clinician in the emotional experiences of their patients facing diseases and death. There is an emotional labour to be borne by the doctor [43].

Other challenges in this kind of work are the risk of non-engagement. The risk is greater where students are compelled to engage in this work, but the gains may also be higher when they do (it may be the people who do not choose this work who need it the most) [44, 45]. Finally this work is time consuming and demanding for educators who may already be hard pressed. On the other hand, it can be meaningful and enriching and thereby an antidote to the risk of cynicism and burnout.

Limitations to the wider application of this work include the fact that it has all been carried out with first and second year students and it may be that disease-centred approaches and cynicism grow in later years of the course [46]. Other limitations include the fact that students were self-selecting in both examples, however such a large number of students were choosing creative enquiry in Example 1 that this course continues now with compulsory creative enquiry. For some students in Example 2, the group work was not their first choice, but where they have written about this, it is to make the point that they were grateful for being placed on this course.

How courses or creative enquiry options are framed for students is important. The work detailed above has all been framed within the practitioner development focus – what would happen if they were optional courses for human flourishing. This is being piloted locally in a different context – for MSc students including those studying on 'Creative arts and mental health' MSc. It has resulted in a small but engaged group of students taking part. We also launched a lockdown creative enquiry group called 'Interpretive voices' in April 2020 spanning medical students, clinicians and academics. This was a space for connection, interpretation and engagement with lived experience and working practice across isolation and disciplinary boundaries. The belief is that flourishing may arise by connecting with 'what is' rather than instructions to 'do better' (eat well, sleep well).

Transferability of the models as presented above may be limited given the resource and time implications; however the creative enquiry essence of space, silence, creative engagement and vulnerable leadership can be introduced in so many ways across the curriculum. Recently a new creative enquiry prize has been initiated locally which invites students to engage creatively and face the climate crisis we are finding ourselves in. This may facilitate dialogue and engagement rather than suppressing the fears and challenges of our times. Other options might include inviting students on placement or as part of a professionalism or flourishing programme to share lived experience and dialogue through a chosen poem or image. The metaphors work powerfully to deepen and personalise reflection [6].

Future research is needed in order to extend our understanding of the contribution creative enquiry can make towards flourishing in medical education, the challenges of embedding and facilitating this work including educator development, and the potential for arts for health or arts therapist engagement in the curriculum. Understanding the challenges as well as impact of creative enquiry programmes on medical culture and the hidden curriculum could act as a catalyst towards more widespread change.

In summary, there is a growing picture in medical education and in clinical practice of stress and burnout. Though there are many possible underlying reasons for this, I have focussed here on features such as the depersonalisation and competition embodied within the undergraduate hidden curriculum, juxtaposed with the emotional burden and complexity of clinical practice. Through medical student engagement in creative enquiry I have found that given the right learning context medical students can engage in different ways of knowing and learning. Where there is a creative and trusting learning environment students share more of their ideas, stories and beliefs. This may lead to rich dialogue, connection and, for some, transformation and growth thereby potentially contributing to eudaimonic flourishing.

Through in-depth practice and research this chapter offers some core constructs to educators interested in developing their human flourishing programmes through creative enquiry. They can be summarised with the acronym *VVV*, that is *Vulnerable leadership, Valuing* and *Voice. Vulnerable leadership* involves the facilitator presenting themselves as human acknowledging the inevitability of our individual inadequacies and collective failings. *Valuing* means inviting awareness of the intrinsic value and shared humanity of both the other and ourselves, whether student, patient or health care professional. Finally *Voice* relates to personal ways of knowing and exploring lived experience, inviting boundary work for the facilitator and students – what to share or keep private, the personal and professional boundaries between patient and future doctor and working across cognitive and emotional boundaries.

In summary, 'people matter'. Creative enquiry practiced as detailed in this chapter, honours the importance for the health care professional of our relationship with *ourselves* as well as that of the *other*.

REFERENCES

1. Scannell, K. (2002). Writing for our lives: physician narratives and medical practice. *Annals of Internal Medicine* 137 (9): 779–781.
2. Cribb, A. and Bignold, S. (1999). Towards the reflexive medical school: the hidden curriculum and medical education research. *Studies in Higher Education* 24: 195–209.
3. Hafferty, F.W. (1998). Beyond curriculum reform: confronting medicine's hidden curriculum. *Academic Medicine* 73 (4): 403–407.
4. Kuper, A. (2007). The intersubjective and the intrasubjective in the patient–physician dyad: implications for medical humanities education. *Medical Humanities* 33 (2): 75–80.

5. Good, B.J. and MJD, G. (1993). Learning medicine. the construction of medical knowledge at harvard medical school. In: *Knowledge, Power and Practice The Anthropology of Medicine and Everyday Life* (eds. S. Lindenbaum and M. Lock), 79–107. California: University of California Press.

6. Younie, L. and Swinglehurst, D. (2019). Creative enquiry and reflective general practice. *The British Journal of General Practice* 69 (686): 446–447.

7. Younie, L. (2019). Vulnerability, resilience and the arts. In: *Body Talk: Whose Language?* (eds. J. Patterson and F. Kinchington), 64–77. Newcastle upon Tyne: Cambridge Scholars.

8. Younie, L. (2006). A qualitative study of the contribution medical humanities can bring to medical education. MSc dissertation. University of Bristol, Bristol.

9. Younie, L. (2011). A reflexive journey through arts-based inquiry in medical education. EdD Dissertation. University of Bristol, Bristol.

10. MacKenzie, S.K. and Wolf, M.M. (2012). Layering sel(f)ves: finding acceptance, community and praxis through collage. *The Qualitative Report* 17 (31): 1–21.

11. Haidet, P., Jarecke, J., Adams, N.E. et al. (2016). A guiding framework to maximise the power of the arts in medical education: a systematic review and metasynthesis. *Medical Education* 50 (3): 320–331.

12. Teodorczuk, A., Thomson, R., Chan, K., and Rogers, G.D. (2017). When I say . . . resilience. *Medical Education* 51 (12): 1206–1208.

13. Shapiro, J., Coulehan, J., Wear, D., and Montello, M. (2009). Medical humanities and their discontents: definitions, critiques, and implications. *Academic Medicine* 84 (2): 192–198.

14. Wright, P. and Pascoe, R. (2015). Eudaimonia and creativity: the art of human flourishing. *Cambridge Journal of Education* 45 (3): 295–306.

15. Dodge, R., Daly, A., and Sanders, L. (2012). The challenge of defining wellbeing. *International Journal of Wellbeing* 2 (3): 222–235.

16. Huta, V. (2015). The complementary roles of eudaimonia and hedonia and how they can be pursued in practice. In: *Positive Psychology in Practice: Promoting Human Flourishing in Work, Health, Education, and Everyday Life* (ed. S. Joseph), 159–182. Wiley.

17. Dyrbye, L.N., Thomas, M.R., and Shanafelt, T.D. (2005). Medical student distress: causes, consequences, and proposed solutions. *Mayo Clinic Proceedings* 80 (12): 1613–1622.

18. Farrell, S., Kadhum, M., Lewis, T. et al. (2019). Wellbeing and burnout amongst medical students in England. *International Review of Psychiatry* 31 (7–8): 579–583.

19. General Medical Council (2019). Caring for doctors, caring for patients: an independent review chaired by Professor Michael West and Dame Denise Coia. https://www.gmc-uk.org/about/how-we-work/corporate-strategy-plans-and-impact/supporting-a-profession-under-pressure/UK-wide-review-of-doctors-and-medical-students-wellbeing

20. British Medical Association (2019). Caring for the mental health of the medical workforce. https://bma.org.uk/collective-voice/policy-and-research/education-training-and-workforce/supporting-the-mental-health-of-doctors-in-the-workforce

21. APPG. All-Party Parliamentary Group on Arts, Health and Wellbeing (2017). Creative Health: The Arts for Health and Wellbeing. *Inquiry Report.*

22. Fancourt, D. and Finn S. 2019. What is the Evidence on the Role of the Arts in Improving Health and Well-Being? A Scoping Review. Health Evidence Network (HEN) synthesis report. World Health Organisation – Europe, Copenhagen. https://www.euro.who.int/en/publications/abstracts/what-is-the-evidence-on-the-role-of-the-arts-in-improving-health-and-well-being-a-scoping-review-2019?fbclid=IwAR3OTYr6Pw0qDL_DY7ISiBR1V0sd6dkiSxYYJVDoaP0Y0gpmOSbJF6c3Los

23. Fancourt, D. and Steptoe, A. (2019). The role of the arts within health. BMJ Opinion.

24. Maudsley, G. and Strivens, J. (2000). Promoting professional knowledge, experiential learning and critical thinking for medical students. *Medical Education* 34 (7): 535–544.

25. Polanyi, M. (1961). Knowing and being. *Mind* 70 (280): 458–470.

26. Younie, L. (2009). Developing narrative competence in medical students. *Medical Humanities* 35 (1): 54.

27. Younie, L. (2013). Introducing arts-based inquiry into medical education: 'exploring the creative arts in health and illness'. In: *Creativity in the Classroom: Case Studies in Using the Arts in Teaching and Learning in Higher Education* (eds. P. McIntosh and D. Warren). Bristol: Intellect Publishers.

28. Younie, L. (2016). Vulnerable leadership. *London Journal of Primary Care* 8 (3): 37–38.

29. Belfiore, M. (1994). The group takes care of itself: art therapy to prevent burnout. *The Arts in Psychotherapy* 21 (2): 119–126.

30. Schei, E. (2006). Doctoring as leadership, the power to heal. *Perspectives in Biology and Medicine* 49 (3): 393–406.

31. Fish, D. (1998). *Practice in the Caring Professions*. Oxford: Butterworth-Heinemann.

32. Younie, L. (2019). Flourishing through creative enquiry London: Queen Mary University of London. https://www.creativeenquiry.qmul.ac.uk/?page_id=213.

33. Hepworth, B. (1970). *A Pictorial Autobiography*. London: Tate Publishing.

34. Csikszentmihalyi, M. (1990). *Flow: The Psychology of Optimal Experience*. New York: Harper and Row.

35. Milligan, E. and Woodley, E. (2009). Creative expressive encounters in health ethics education: teaching ethics as relational engagement. *Teaching and Learning in Medicine: An International Journal* 21 (2): 131–139.

36. Elliott, B. (2011). Arts-based and narrative inquiry in liminal experience reveal platforming as basic social psychological process. *The Arts in Psychotherapy* 38: 96–103.

37. Bub, B. (2006). *Communication Skills that Heal: A Practical Approach to a New Professionalism in Medicine*. Oxford: Radcliffe Publishing.

38. Tharenos, C.L., Hayden, A.M., and Cook, E. (2019). Resident self-portraiture: a reflective tool to explore the journey of becoming a doctor. *The Journal of Medical Humanities* 40 (4): 529–551.

39. Satici, S.A., Uysal, R., and Akin, A. (2013). Investigating the relationship between flourishing and self-compassion: a structural equation modeling approach. *Psychologica Belgica* 53 (4): 85–99.

40. Lee Roze des Ordons, A., de Groot, J.M., Rosenal, T. et al. (2018). How clinicians integrate humanism in their clinical workplace-'Just trying to put myself in their human being shoes'. *Perspectives on Medical Education* 7 (5): 318–324.

41. Haidet, P. (2007). Jazz and the 'art' of medicine: improvisation in the medical encounter. *Annals of Family Medicine* 5 (2): 164–169.

42. Seeley, C. (2011). Uncharted territory: imagining a stronger relationship between the arts and action research. *Action Research* 9 (1): 83–99.

43. Kerasidou, A. and Horn, R. (2016). Making space for empathy: supporting doctors in the emotional labour of clinical care. *BMC Medical Ethics* 17: 8.

44. Thompson, T., Lamont-Robinson, C., and Younie, L. (2010). 'Compulsory creativity': rationales, recipes, and results in the placement of mandatory creative endeavour in a medical undergraduate curriculum. *Medical Education Online* 15: 5394. https://doi.org/10.3402/meo.v15i0.5394, http://www.med-ed-online.net/index.php/meo/article/view/5394.

45. Kirklin, D., Meakin, R., Singh, S., and Lloyd, M. (2000). Living with and dying from cancer: a humanities special study module. *Medical Humanities* 26 (1): 51–54.

46. Hojat, M., Vergare, M.J., Maxwell, K. et al. (2009). The devil is in the third year: a longitudinal study of erosion of empathy in medical school. *Academic Medicine* 84: 1182–1191.

CHAPTER 3

Embracing Difference

Towards an Understanding of Queer Identities in Medicine

Helen Bintley[1] and Jo Winning[2]

[1] Barts and The London School of Medicine and Dentistry, Queen Mary University of London, London, UK

[2] Department of English, Theatre and Creative Writing, Birkbeck, University of London, London, UK

CONTEXT

Locating the Problem

Members of LGBTQ+ communities experience poorer physical and mental health than those in heterosexual communities [1–4].[1] Data concerning the extent of these healthcare inequalities is limited and often not robust, particularly in relation to trans communities [2].[2] However, discrimination appears to play a significant part in perpetuating these health inequalities creating, barriers to treatment and preventing access to screening tests [5, 6].

As well as affecting health, discrimination affects LGBTQ+ identifying people in a variety of other social contexts including employment. For instance, a recent British Medical Association GLADD (the association of LGBTQ+ doctors and dentists) survey of LGB identifying doctors in the United Kingdom found 70% had experienced some sort of homophobia or biphobia and more than 1 in 10 had experienced harassment or discrimination in the workplace in the last two years [7]. This discrimination, when paired with studies (although few in number) that suggest that healthcare professionals have poor overall health due to their occupation [8–11], makes LGBTQ+ identifying healthcare professionals a group potentially vulnerable to mental and physical ill health.

To start to tackle the discrimination experienced by this group, we argue that we need to think in more nuanced ways about identity and difference.[3] In medicine, the 'body', in all its diversity, is an embodied entity that is utilised, marginalised and categorised by stakeholders to control and enact agendas. The language used to create categories in this context has the propensity to compartmentalise people into, for instance, 'male or female', ignoring the complexity of gender identities between and within these categories. Language-use within medicine has the capacity both to create norms and to occlude those who sit 'outside' its categories. The marginalising possibilities of language therefore need to be exposed and challenged. In this chapter the authors co-construct an analysis of embodied difference, drawing on critical frameworks from their seemingly disparate specialities of humanities and medicine.[4]

Following recent methodological advances in medical humanities [12–15], which demonstrate that having a deep understanding of medical culture and practice is only possible through transdisciplinary critical frameworks from across and outside of academic institutions, we bring our different disciplines together to address the experience of LGBTQ+ healthcare practitioners. In doing so, we aim to make visible the complexity of queerness in a medical context and consider ways to reduce discrimination for this group.

In what follows Bintley and Winning describe different language-based approaches they have used to explore queer identity in healthcare and give a voice to this marginalised community. Although different, what our approaches have in common is the utilisation of underlying concepts drawn from the academic fields of queer theory, post-structuralism and intersectional theory. These concepts allow us to excavate otherwise hidden aspects of the lived experience of LGBTQ+ healthcare practitioners.

Being a Body

It is commonplace in medical humanities discussions of clinical practice to understand the clinical gaze as the embodiment of a scopic movement that runs in one direction only, from the clinician to the patient. In his seminal formulation, Michel Foucault describes 'the loquacious gaze' of the clinician, which fixes the body of the patient and her disease in a '*spacialization* and *verbalization* of the pathological' [16, p. xii]. This gaze bespeaks clinical power, it enables the clinician 'to see and to say', thus to observe and diagnose. By implication, the patient's body becomes an object to be examined and defined, irrespective of the nuances of embodied experience and personal affective reality.

However, it is also important to fold in the nuance of Foucault's account of the power relations embedded in the clinical encounter. In his exploration of the discourses that construct human sexuality, Foucault identifies a rather more complex dimension of clinical power that might at first be occluded in the model of the gaze. Power functions not on its own, but works together with a twinned 'mechanism', which is to say, pleasure [17, p. 45]. For the clinician, the exercise of scopic and diagnostic power brings pleasure, but simultaneously there is another kind of pleasure for the patient, that which 'kindles at having to evade this power, flee from it, fool it or travesty it' [17, p. 45]. Here we start to glimpse a patient's agency. Moreover, Foucault's mathematical metaphor for the clinical relationship between 'doctors and patients' is the spiral, in which power and pleasure, observer and observee, circle in continuous movement around each other, co-constituting subjectivities and experiences. What we wish to extract from this complex Foucauldian model is the conceptual purchase it affords us to make visible the often occluded object in the clinical encounter – the clinician's own body.

Understanding the clinician's body as an object both fixed and made vulnerable by the multiple gazes of institutional and regulatory power, as well as those of the patients whose care depends upon it (and the network of other caring bodies with which it works) is a crucial critical move in the framework of this chapter. The increasing attention on the clinician's body, in the face of national (and indeed international) crises of physician burnout, workplace stress and rising suicide rates, is perhaps evidenced best by recent reviews such as Keith Pearson's *NHS Staff and Learners' Mental Wellbeing Commission* [18] and Michael West and Denise Coia's *Caring for doctors, caring for patients: how to transform UK healthcare environments to support doctors and medical students to care for patients* [19].

In their much-anticipated 2019 report West and Coia argue that 'medicine is a tough job, but we make it far harder than it should be by neglecting the simple basics in caring for doctors' wellbeing' [19, p. 12]. Our argument is that such 'simple basics' must not be so simple as to omit difference, to the lived experience of those bodies, which occupy culturally 'peripheral' locations by dint of ethnicity, class or sexual identity.

'Unspeakable Things Unspoken': Linguistic Vulnerability and the Body

In her 1988 Tanner lecture, the African–American novelist and academic Toni Morrison describes the processes by which constructions of an American literary canon (meaning the body of texts and writers highly valued by a culture and seen as the core of a literary tradition) has systematically excluded African–American voices, from the slave narratives of eighteenth and nineteenth centuries to the contemporary writers of the late twentieth century. Such exclusions make it very hard for an oppressed community to speak of their experience since, as Morrison identifies, 'cultures, whether silenced or monologistic, whether repressed or repressing, seek meaning in the language and images available to them' [20, p. 132].

We wish to draw on Morrison's model of the structural relationship between language, identity and exclusion as we consider the lived experience of LGBTQ+ identifying doctors in the United Kingdom. Further, from the panoply of theorizations available across literary theory, feminism and queer theory, we deploy Judith Butler's delineations of linguistic vulnerability and sociality as key concepts to articulate the hidden exclusions experienced by this group.

Bodies, Butler argues, are made possible by and through language. 'Language', she writes, 'sustains the body not by bringing it into being or feeding it in a literal way' but rather by 'being interpolated within the terms of language [so] that a certain social existence of the body first becomes possible' [21, p. 3]. In other words, a body cannot exist, in social terms, without being addressed and described in words that, by common agreement, make sense to other people. Names 'inaugurate and sustain linguistic existence' Butler argues, they 'confer singularity in location and time' [21, pp. 29–30].

To make these potentially abstract pronouncements more concrete, she gives the example that 'there appears to be no "Peter" without the name, "Peter"' [21, p. 32]. This is no simple matter since, as Butler describes, language 'can also threaten its existence' [21, p. 3]. Such threats are found in hate speech, or in the practice of derogation against certain kinds of people or groups, such as in the long, cross-cultural histories of homo- or transphobia. The fact of 'injurious speech' makes human subjects prone to 'linguistic vulnerability', in which name-calling and their corrosive opposites, silence and exclusion (the refusal to give someone a name), impact upon the very *possibility* of existence [21, p. 2].

To consider the impact of linguistic vulnerability within the experience of LGBTQ+ clinicians, we take the recent bestselling memoir *This Is Going To Hurt: The Secret Diaries of a Junior Doctor* by the British comedian and ex-clinician Adam Kay. The written form of Kay's reworked e-portfolio recollections provides a compelling example of the ways in which LGBTQ+ sexual identity becomes unspeakable in the clinical setting. From the outset, Kay's text is riven with allusions to the sexual body. A newly-qualified House Officer is 'a one-man, mobile, essentially untrained A&E department, getting drenched in bodily fluids (not even the fun kind)' [22, p. 6].

Kay's clinical vignettes from his early foundation years, through to his chosen specialty of Obstetrics and Gynaecology, often involve sexual endeavours that have gone awry: 'Less than a year as a doctor and this is the fourth object I have removed from a rectum – professionally at least' [22, p. 22]. The seemingly throwaway quip, in the context of multiple narratives of sexual behaviours that land patients in A&E, is a rare allusion to Kay's own sexuality which is otherwise rendered invisible throughout what is principally a raucous shock-narrative that seeks to 'expose' the visceral traumas of clinical practice.

Kay's own intimate, domestic arrangements are only ever obliquely referenced in the memoir. His partner 'H' is anonymised in a footnote as 'my short-suffering partner of six months' and minimised in importance with the follow-up remark: 'don't worry – you're not going to have to remember huge numbers of characters. It's not *Game of Thrones*', [22, p. 7]. Whilst 'H' is referenced periodically, as Kay's home life becomes relegated to a subsidiary place, H's sex and name are never spoken. More than simply an act of authorial protection of an intimate relationship, this refusal to name is a protective mechanism in the face of linguistic vulnerability. Kay strips his narrative of personal detail, foregrounding patient stories whilst covering the traces of his own. We only learn that his relationship with 'H' has broken down in a glibly short diary entry:

> *Was meant to be back home at 7 p.m. sharp but it's 9.30 and I've only just come off labour ward. Feels appropriate that work commitments mean I have to reschedule collecting all my belongings from the flat. On the plus side, my depressing new bachelor pad is only ten minutes from the hospital [22, p. 252].*

From a literary studies perspective, there is a striking contradiction in Kay's occlusion of his own sexual identity in a text constructed to appeal to a lay audience's strong desire to 'see behind' the alluring, 'shocking' world of clinical practice. Yet when read in the context of medical culture, the desire to 'hide' the name of his sexual identity is highly legible as self-protection. As we have argued earlier in this chapter, the patient's gaze, alongside that of the institutional and regulatory gazes of medical culture and governance, do their own repressive work on the clinician's body. In interviews given at the time of increasing public interest in his memoir, Kay most commonly utilizes deflective humour to shift the conversation away from his sexuality. As the journalist Karl Webster notes in his 2017 interview, 'Kay describes himself as not "mega-comfortable" talking about his sexuality' [23].

Kay's fame (at the time of writing this chapter, the second volume of his memoir, *Twas the Nightshift Before Christmas* charted immediately on publication) has generated much public discussion on social media platforms. Following Butler's explanation of the power of naming, and the linguistic vulnerability of the LGBTQ+ clinician, many of these public discussions about Kay 'fill in' the identity of the long-suffering 'H' in his memoir as a female partner, 'his then-girlfriend whose identity has been protected' [24]. This projection of heterosexual sexual identity into the linguistic vacuum left by Kay's self-protective refusal to name it, evidences the terrain we map in this chapter, in which difference remains unspoken and the clinician's body becomes a site constructed by patient assumptions and the 'normativity' promoted by regulatory discourses.

DESCRIPTION

Challenging Values and Questioning Norms: The Medical Curriculum as Discourse

Core to medical practice is the understanding of people, their bodies and the impact of clinicians and their practice on these elements of human experience. Where concepts such as the clinical gaze or the agency of clinicians opens up a deeper critical understanding of the clinical encounter, we argue that it is important to understand and make visible the myriad of complex, intersecting factors of identity within the clinical encounter, including gender and sexuality. Appreciating how these factors apply to interactions between the embodied individuals in the encounter highlight the difficulties within and between such relationships.

Moreover, we can see that language, or the lack of it, plays a large part in socially-constructed understandings of bodies in many contexts, including health-care. Key to our understanding of medical practice, education and culture in this chapter is the Foucauldian concept of discourse, in which 'power and knowledge are joined together' [17, p. 100]. Epitomised by socio-cultural domains such as law, religion and medicine, discourse is defined as 'bodies of ideas that produce and regulate the world in their own terms, rendering some things commonplace and other things nonsensical' [25, p. 36]. In the following analysis we consider the medical curriculum as an example of Foucauldian discourse that foregrounds het-erosexuality as a normative sexual identity and at best occludes, or at worst pathol-ogises LGBTQ+ identity. In the following discussion, we examine an empirical example from our research that explores expressions of queer identity (and identity more generally) amongst those involved in medical education. We explore the chal-lenges faced by professionals when talking about identity in the medical context and consider the implications of such challenges for undergraduate medical cur-ricula in the UK.[5]

The research question which structured Bintley's study considered how power, language and discourse impact upon medical education professionals' understand-ings of LGBTQ+ people and how these understandings, or lack of them, aid or hinder the development of curricula and conversations around difference. The methodolog-ical framework for this study is based upon Feminist Post-structural Discourse Anal-ysis (*FPDA*) [26]. Judith Baxter's model of FPDA brings together post-structuralism and feminism, two bodies of thought which have been critical of each other, in order to create a 'productive contradiction' that allows us to develop a deeper critical under-standing of each approach. This productive contradiction can then be utilised to transform our understanding of subjects. In the context of medical education, we might assume that the inclusion of notions of diversity enhances the visibility of, and linguistic fluency around, identity and difference. However, there is evidence that educational diversity interventions in healthcare perpetuate the categorisation, mar-ginalisation and silencing of diverse people [27, 28].

Sixteen participants were recruited to the study from professional services, aca-demia and senior management, by stratified sampling, in one medical school in the UK. Three multi-task focus groups were undertaken with each of the three professional groups. Each focus group had three parts; a facilitated introductory discussion about the curriculum and LGBTQ+ identity, a group activity around LGBTQ+ curriculum development and a peer-led debrief. The focus groups were video recorded to analyse both verbal and non-verbal language and an inductive approach was used to under-take denotative and connotative analyses in line with FPDA. Following iterative cycles of analysis over a 12-month period, three discourses were identified: comfort, hierarchy and expectation

The results illustrated that participants felt uncomfortable talking about gender and sexuality because they felt that they were uninformed about these elements of identity. As in Kay's memoir, no one openly discussed their own gender identity or sexual orientation. In addition, participants felt that students were better informed about some LGBTQ+ issues than they were. The participants related this discomfort to a general lack of conversation about health and illness amongst healthcare and healthcare education professionals, noting that poor mental and physical health amongst doctors was not discussed in the curriculum enough. Even so, the participants highlighted the need for staff development so that they could have a language to start conversations about these issues.

The results also suggested that established hierarchies were both important for curriculum development and also disempowering. This was linked to the participants' perception of a rigid, top-down approach, in which senior managers were most powerful and professional services staff were least powerful. Within this, participants understood expectations of themselves and the medical curriculum as complex, dynamic and challenging. These expectations were associated with power and gender, and the curriculum was seen as either a transactional process or as an embodied entity with power of its own.

The outcomes of this study highlight the impact of power, language and discourse on medical education professionals' ability to challenge established norms and discuss queer identity with staff and students. Although only carried out in one institution, and therefore not generalisable, these findings support other research which suggests the strong and urgent need for curriculum change in this respect [27, 29, 30]. In the final section we consider how change may be enacted by considering the potential of productive contradictions [26] such as intersectionality and transdisciplinarity [31] in transforming our conversations with about identity and difference in healthcare.

FUTURE DIRECTIONS

Towards Change

We have seen so far that if we want to consider linguistic and theoretical understandings of the body, health and illness in the context of healthcare inequality we need to think beyond the established norms and understand the body as marked by difference. Applying theory to practice, in this section we explore future possibilities for health inequality research and the kinds of concepts that advance understandings of the queer body and health. By writing as a collaborative team across disciplines we aim to demonstrate an empirical example of transdisciplinary working and the power of such a collaboration in transforming our understanding of queer identity in medical education.

We have seen that language and discourse play a large part in socially-constructed understandings of bodies in many contexts, including healthcare. Cultural narratives about discourse related to health and illness are as varied as language itself and are imbued with power, which influences our understanding of peoples' bodies. Cultural theories are a way of exposing the entanglements involved in conceptions of health and illness and, more importantly, how we can enact change. Cultural theories span the entirety of culture, space, place and time and depending on the lens adopted, give different insights into the conceptualisation of embodiment and being.

As one example of such theories, in this chapter so far we have explored poststructuralist notions of power and discourse and applied this not only to patient agency but also the embodiment of clinicians. Another example is intersectionality, a term first coined by the critical race theorist Crenshaw [32] to describe the complexity of identity and the double oppressions of racism and sexism experienced by African-American women. Intersectionality enables us to understand the discrimination someone experiences as a consequence of layers of oppression related to interconnected factors such as race, ethnicity, gender and sexuality. Crenshaw [32] describes the impact of discriminating against these component parts of a person's identity and the resultant, multiplicated layers of oppression and discrimination that can occur as a consequence.

What capacity does the concept of intersectionality have to make overt the complexity of peoples' experience of their bodies by highlighting the problematic nature of their objectification in a clinical context. Intersectionality is an important lens through which to view policy and practice and we argue it is a powerful concept for healthcare education, facilitating clinicians' understandings of their own bodies as well as those of their patients. Intersectional understandings have not been fully utilised as educational approaches in healthcare. As a practical consequence, existing educational models do not always challenge stereotypes or discuss the complexity of embodied experiences of patients and healthcare professionals [31].

Moreover, we note that education alone cannot change inherent societal norms such as heteronormativity, an ideological frame that affects people both within and outside of a medical context. Heteronormativity, described by Jeppesen [33] as a societal understanding of relationships in which the perceived dominant structure is heterosexuality, is arguably inherent in healthcare and creates marginalization of LGBTQ+ patients and clinicians alike [34]. To lever this framework open, queer theory provides depth analysis to expose its workings.

Butler [35] argues that heteronormativity creates a 'heterosexual matrix' in which those that do not identify as heterosexual are made 'other'. The matrix constructs heterosexuality as the dominant form of human sexual identity and designates other sexual identities as deviant. In terms resonant to healthcare, the doctor and philosopher Georges Canguilhem describes such power structures as making categories of 'the normal and the pathological' [36], proposing a binary opposition we find useful in our research for exposing the 'norms' imposed around sexual orientation and gender identity within medical culture and education.

What becomes apparent from our research and that of others is that meaningful, effective conversation about identity is missing in medicine and medical education. We argue that having a language to talk about queer bodies is important in facilitating discussions about difficulty and providing healthcare professionals with the tools to reduce healthcare discrimination.

We propose that one way of doing this could be to utilise the 'productive contradictions' of different approaches, just as Baxter [26] does in her construction of the FPDA methodology. As an example, Bintley and George [31] discuss the possibility of utilising the productive contradiction of intersectionality and transdisciplinarity to facilitate education and conversation related to difference. As we note above, the first of these concepts is drawn from critical race studies and has become a common theoretical concept for making visible the multiple factors of identity. The second concept constitutes a radical methodological approach which, as the theoretical physicist Nicolescu [37–39] writes, incorporates thinking and research 'which is at once between the disciplines, across the disciplines and beyond the disciplines . . . one of the imperatives is the unity of knowledge' [39, p. 187]. Nicolescu outlines the transformative possibilities of thinking beyond single, bounded disciplines for embracing the complexity found in the space between them.

Drawing these two terms together creates productive friction. Intersectionality seeks to explore issues within social systems in a way that Nicolescu [39] would argue is restrictive for knowledge creation. Conversely, other schools of transdisciplinarity have argued that Nicolescu's approach is too abstract and is not directly applicable to world issues [40]. However, these contradictions can be productive. For instance, on the one hand the feminist sociological frame of intersectional theory would seem closed off to other modes of thought. On the other, the model of transdisciplinarity, which seems to overlook the hierarchy of disciplines (think of the current inequity between the arts and humanities disciplines and those of science, medicine and technology), seems closed off to structures of power and difference. Yet both terms, when brought together, contribute much-needed groundedness to the other.

As such Bintley and George argue that intersectional transdisciplinarity (*ISTD*) could be a useful methodology for understanding difference in the healthcare setting. Bintley and George define ISTD in relation to difference as, 'striv[ing] for unity of knowledge about existence that utilises perspectives from across, between and beyond disciplines in relation to inequality, inequity and oppression outside of the constraints of isolated social systems' [31]. ISTD then has the potential to demonstrate the complexity of difference and in so doing aid medical education professionals and clinicians in starting conversations about their own bodies and those of others.

The collaborative writing approach in this chapter may well be described as intersectional transdisciplinarity. We write as scholars and experts in disparate fields but also as patients, and observers of the clinical encounter. The different approaches we bring to understanding complex clinical interactions, using literary materials alongside cultural theory and empirical research, changes both our perspectives on the lived experiences of clinicians' and patients' bodies and makes clear the inequalities and occlusions present within clinical encounters.

Yet we also recognize that embracing difference within medical culture requires an intersectional awareness of socio-political factors. We argue that it is vital to consider difference, and its associated inequalities, on micro-, meso- and macro-societal levels in order to change perspectives and attitudes. To do this, methods of marginalised voices being heard need to be utilised in a way that does not descend into politically-driven, tick-box exercises. National and international policy, political activism and technology are all ways in which embodied difference could be discussed more effectively in the future. However, with all these approaches needs to come an understanding of the importance of contradiction and conflict and the transformative possibilities of conversation in spite of, and because of, these elements. In this way, the messiness of who we are, what we are and who we might become is simultaneously embraced, rejected and re-considered. Only through this difficult process will conversations and collaborations change the status quo.

NOTES

1. LGBTQ+ refers to Lesbian, Gay, Bisexual, Transgender, Queer and other identifying sexual minorities in this chapter. The history of terms used to describe sexual identity is long and complex. In the strong spirit of inclusion, the authors adopt this common initialism to gesture to the many and varied human sexual identities. The other term in use in this chapter, queer, similarly works inclusively to describe sexual identities and desires located outside the normative model of heterosexuality.

2. We take our definition of trans from the Stonewall glossary that being, 'An umbrella term to describe people whose gender is not the same as, or does not sit comfortably with, the sex they were assigned at birth' (https://www.stonewall.org.uk/help-advice/glossary-terms) (accessed 23 April 2020).

3. We take the term 'difference' from the fields of feminist, black and queer scholarship, which is used to define those identities other than the dominant subject (white, heterosexual and male) of mainstream Western culture. For a seminal delineation of this work, see Audre Lorde's chapter 'Age, Race, Class, and Sex: Women Redefining Difference' in her *Sister Outsider* (Berkeley, CA: The Crossing Press, 1984).

4. Embodied difference here refers to the way that bodies and bodily experience are marked by factors of identity such as non-normative sexual identity.

5. This empirical research was undertaken in the course of HB's Masters' thesis and is included in this publication with the consent of the participants.

REFERENCES

1. Boehmer, U., Miao, W., Maxwell, N., and Ozonoff, A. (2014). Sexual minority population density and incidence of lung, colorectal and female breast cancer in California. *BMJ Open* 4 (3): 1–7.

2. Hudson-Sharp, N. and Metcalf, H. (2016). *Inequality Among Lesbian, Gay, Bisexual and Transgender Groups in the UK: A Review of Evidence*. London: NIESR.

3. Reisner, S.L., Poeat, T., Keatley, J. et al. (2016). Global health burden and needs of transgender populations: a review. *Lancet* 388: 412–436.

4. Muller, A. (2017). Scrambling for access: availability, accessibility, acceptability and quality of healthcare for lesbian, gay, bisexual and transgender people in South Africa. *BMC International Health and Human Rights* 17: 16. https://doi.org/10.1186/s12914-017-0124-4.

5. Fish, J. and Bewley, S. (2010). Using human rights-based approaches to conceptualise lesbian and bisexual women's health inequality. *Health & Social Care in the Community* 18 (4): 355–362.

6. Ceres, M., Quinn, G.P., Loscalzo, M., and Rice, D. (2018). Cancer screening considerations and cancer screening uptake for LGBT persons. *Seminars in Oncology Nursing* 34 (1): 37–51.

7. BMA (2016). The experience of lesbian, gay and bisexual doctors in the NHS: discrimination in the workplace or place of study. https://www.bma.org.uk/media/1094/bma_experience-of-lgb-doctors-and-medical-students-in-nhs-oct-2019.pdf (accessed 10 October 2019).

8. Aagestad, C., Tyssen, R., and Sterud, T. (2016). Do work-related factors contribute to differences in doctor-certified sick leave? A prospective study comparing women in health and social occupations with women in the general work population. *BMC Public Health* 16: 235. https://doi.org/10.1186/s12889-016-2908-1.

9. Smith, F., Goldacre, M.J., and Lambert, T.W. (2017). Adverse effects on health and wellbeing of working as a doctor: views of the UK medical graduates of 1974 and 1977 surveyed in 2014. *Journal of the Royal Society of Medicine* 110 (5): 198–207.

10. Milner, A., King, T.L., and Kavanagh, A. (2019). The mental health impacts of health and human service work: longitudinal evidence about differential exposure and susceptibility using 16 waves of cohort data. *Preventive Medicine Reports* 14: 100826. https://doi.org/10.1016/j.pmedr.2019.100826.

11. GMC (2019). National Training surveys, Initial findings report. https://www.gmc-uk.org/-/media/documents/national-training-surveys-initial-findings-report-2019_pdf-84390391.pdf (accessed August 2019).

12. Macnaughton, J. (2011). Medical humanities challenge to medicine. *Journal of Evaluation in Clinical Practice* 17 (5): 927–932.

13. Fitzgerald, D. and Callard, F. (2016). Entangling the medical humanities. In: *The Edinburgh Companion to the Critical Medical Humanities* (eds. A. Woods and A. Whitehead), 35–49. Edinburgh: Edinburgh University Press.

14. Chiavaroli, N. (2017). Knowing how we know: an epistemological rationale for the medical humanities. *Medical Education* 51: 13–21.

15. Winning, J. (2018). Learning to think-with: feminist epistemology and the practice-based Medical Humanities. *Feminist Encounters* 2 (2): 20. https://doi.org/10.20897/femenc/3888.

16. Foucault, M. (2007). *The Birth of the Clinic: An Archeology of Medical Perception*. London and New York: Routledge.

17. Foucault, M. (1980). *The History of Sexuality: An Introduction*, vol. 1. New York: Vintage.

18. Pearson, K. (2019). NHS staff and learners, Mental Wellbeing Commission. Health Education England. https://www.hee.nhs.uk/sites/default/files/documents/NHS%20 (HEE)%20-%20Mental%20Wellbeing%20Commission%20Report.pdf (accessed 23 December 2020).

19. West, M. and Coia, D. (2019). Caring for doctors, caring for patients: how to transform UK healthcare environments to support doctors and medical students to care for patients. https://www.gmc-uk.org/-/media/documents/caring-for-doctors-caring-for-patients_pdf-80706341.pdf (accessed 23 December 2019).

20. Morrison, T. (1988). Unspeakable things unspoken: the Afro-American presence in American literature. The Tanner lecture on Human values. https://tannerlectures. utah.edu/_documents/a-to-z/m/morrison90.pdf (accessed 23 December 2019).

21. Butler, J. (1997). *Excitable Speech: A politics of the Performative*. London and New York: Routledge.

22. Kay, A. (2017). *This is Going to Hurt: The Secret Diaries of a Junior Doctor*. London: Picador.

23. Webster, K. (2017). A Lehrer, Lehrer Laughs: Adam Kay and the Remains of Tom Lehrer. https://karlwebster.com/adam_kay_tom_lehrer.

24. Crawford, F. (2017). Review of 'this is going to hurt'. The Boomerange Books Blog. https://blog.boomerangbooks.com.au/review-going-hurt-secret-diaries-junior-doctor/2017/10 (accessed 10 December 2020).

25. Youdell, D. (2006). Diversity, inequality, and a post-structural politics for education. *Discourse: Studies in the Cultural Politics of Education* 27 (1): 33–42.

26. Baxter, J. (2003). *Positioning Gender in Discourse: A Feminist Methodology*. London: Palgrave MacMillon.

27. Dogra, N., Bhatti, F., Ertubey, C. et al. (2015). Teaching diversity to medical undergraduate; curriculum development, delivery and assessment: AMEE guide no. 103. *Medical Teacher* 38 (4): 323–337.

28. Sorensen, J., Norredam, M., Surrmond, J. et al. (2019). Need for ensuring cultural competence in medical programmes of European universities. *BMC Medical Education* 19 (21): 1–8.

29. Obedin-Maliver, J., Goldsmith, E.S., Stewart, L. et al. (2011). Lesbian, gay, bisexual and transgender-related content in undergraduate medical education. *Journal of the American Medical Association* 306 (9): 971–977.

30. Parameshwaran, V., Cockbain, B.C., Hillyeard, M., and Price, J.R. (2017). Is the lack of specific lesbian, gay, bisexual, transgender and queer/ questioning (LGBTQ) health care education in medical school a cause for concern? Evidence from a survey of knowledge and practice among UK medical students. *Journal of Homosexuality* 64 (3): 367–381.

31. Bintley, H. and George, R.E. (2020). Teaching diversity in healthcare education: conceptual clarity and the need for an intersectional transdisciplinary approach. In: *Clinical Education for the Health Professions* (eds. D. Nestel, G. Reedy, L. McKenna and S. Gough). Singapore: Springer.

32. Crenshaw, K. (1990). Mapping the margins: intersectionality, identity politics, and violence against women of color. *Stanford Law Review* 43 (6): 1241–1299.

33. Jeppesen, S. (2016). Heteronormativity. In: *The SAGE Encyclopedia of LGBTQ Studies* (ed. A.E. Goldberg), 493–496. Thousand Oaks, CA: SAGE Publishing.

34. Pallotta-Chiaroll, M. and Martin, E. (2009). 'Which sexuality? which service?': bisexual young people's experience with youth, queer and mental health services in Australia. *Journal of LGBT Youth* 6 (2–3): 199–222.

35. Butler, J. (1990). *Gender Trouble: Feminism and the Subversion of Identity*. New York: Routledge.

36. Canguilhem, G. (1991). *The Normal and the Pathological*. New York: Zone Books.

37. Nicolescu, B. (2002). *Manifesto of Transdisciplinarity*. New York: SUNY Press.

38. Nicolescu, B. (2006). Transdisciplinarity—Past, Present and Future. In: *Moving World-Views—Reshaping Sciences, Policies and Practices for Endogenous Sustainable Development* (eds. B. Haverkort and C. Reijntjes), 142–166. Amsterdam, Holland: COMPAS Editions.

39. Nicolescu, B. (2014). Methodology of transdisciplinarity. World Futures: *The Journal of New Paradigm Research* 70 (3–4): 186–199.

40. Gibbons, M., Limoges, C., Nowotny, H. et al. (1994). *The New Production of Knowledge*. London: Sage.

CHAPTER 4

Stress and Mental Well-Being in Emergency Medical Dispatchers

Astrid Coxon

Institute of Psychiatry, Psychology & Neuroscience, King's College London, London, UK

CONTEXT

When a member of the public contacts emergency medical services (*EMS*) in the UK, their call is processed via a regional Emergency Operations Centre (*EOC*). Initially, the call is managed by a call operative, who records information relevant to the emergency, including details of the patient's condition. Using a triaging system (such as National Health Service [*NHS*] Pathways), the call handler processes this information to categorise the severity of the emergency. These details are then passed to a member of the ambulance dispatch team (also referred to as emergency medical dispatchers or simply dispatchers). The dispatchers manage available EMS resources (ambulances) and dispatch them appropriately based on location, availability and medical need.

Being the first point of contact for members of the public needing EMS support puts EOC staff under considerable stress and pressure. This, added to long and often unsociable hours, understaffing and a lack of appropriate support, has been blamed for ever-increasing staff sickness absence in the emergency medical sector [1–3]. The latest sickness absence report from the UK Office for National Statistics (ONS) stated a national average sickness rate of 2.5% for women and 1.6% for men [4], a rate which has steadily decreased over the past 16 years [5]. However, sickness absence rates for UK NHS staff are higher than in the rest of the UK workforce, rising from 3.8% in 2018 to 4.1% in 2019 [6], with nearly a quarter of absences attributed to stress, anxiety, depression or other mental health issues. Sickness absence in EMS workers is higher still, with up to a

The Mental Health and Wellbeing of Healthcare Practitioners: Research and Practice, First Edition.
Edited by Esther Murray and Jo Brown.
© 2021 John Wiley & Sons Ltd. Published 2021 by John Wiley & Sons Ltd.

third taking time off due to stress [7]. This high rate of stress-related sickness absence could be attributed to role-specific stressors, such as exposure to trauma, working long and often erratic shift patterns and the life-saving, time-limited work undertaken.

Despite the recognised issue of stress-related sickness absence in EMS staff, there is currently limited published research in this area, compared to other healthcare professionals such as ward nurses [8–10] and surgeons [11–13]. Of the limited EMS literature available, the focus is largely on frontline staff such as emergency room nurses, paramedics and ambulance technicians [14–17]. It is largely recognised that these roles are inherently stressful due to exposure to trauma and distress, having to take life-saving action and the demands of time-limited working with limited resources. The short- and long-term health implications have been well-documented and proposals for support interventions proposed.

But what of the EOC staff 'behind the scenes'? Integral to the working of EMS are those staff members who take emergency calls, offer immediate telephone support, and manage available resources to dispatch ambulances and paramedics to emergencies appropriately. Whilst there is a growing body of research which explores the stress and psychological well-being of office-based EMS staff [3, 17–21], the lived experiences of ambulance dispatch staff is largely undocumented in academic literature. Looking at the broader literature, such as research into stress experienced by dispatchers in other emergency services, offers further insights. Law enforcement research demonstrates a similar pattern as that of EMS: frontline workers have been highly studied, but dispatch personnel have received little attention [22]. However, this research does suggest that particular attention should be paid to unique intra- and inter-person stressors experienced by dispatch staff. In their theoretical framework of stress and work, Payne and Fletcher highlight that both extra-person stressors (such as work environment) and intra-person stressors (such as feelings of guilt) can both contribute to psychological and physiological strain which, if unaddressed, can develop into a chronic state of stress [23, 24]. Existing EMS research largely focuses on extra-person and organisational stressors [20, 25], highlighting the need for intra-person stressors (and the strategies dispatchers employ to manage these) to be explored in the present study.

In this chapter, I describe a qualitative study conducted at an EOC in the south of England [26]. This study provides an in-depth exploration of the stress experienced by ambulance dispatchers in an NHS setting, how they feel stress affects them and their work, and how they currently manage work-related stress. The chapter concludes by exploring potential strategies for managing stress related to EOC work and proposing directions for future research.

DESCRIPTION

To explore how ambulance dispatchers experienced work-related stress, nine ambulance dispatchers were interviewed about their role and the stress they experienced. Participants (five male, four female) were purposefully recruited from a

population of 36 permanent staff at an EOC in the south of England. All nine participants identified as white British and were aged between 26 and 60 years. Two of the
nine participants had previous medical training (as first aiders) before joining the
EOC. Participants' experience in their current role ranged from 2 to 14 years.

Participants were interviewed individually and face-to-face, following a semi-
structured interview schedule. This interview schedule was developed in consultation
with the EOC manager and my colleagues, with reference to existing literature, to
ensure that relevant topics were covered and pertinent questions asked. The key topics
covered their motivations for working in the EOC, the stress they encountered in the
role and their mechanisms/strategies for managing stress.

Participants were asked:

1. Tell me a little about your role – when did you first decide to work in emergency
   dispatch centre (*EDC*)?
   a. Why did you decide to work in EDC? What attracted you?
   b. What were your expectations – were those met? How and why?
   c. Is there anything about the job that surprised you – good or bad? Anything
      you did not expect?
2. What do you find rewarding about working in EDC?
   a. Is there a particular aspect of the job you enjoy? (Prompts: The job itself,
      the team and the type of work?)
   b. What are your key motivators for going to work?
3. Can you give me an example of a particularly difficult or stressful incident you
   have dealt with whilst working in EDC?
   a. What happened? (Prompts: Describe the event unfolding.)
   b. What about it was difficult or stressful? What made it different from your
      usual incidents?
   c. How did you deal with the incident? (Prompts: During the incident.
      Immediately after the incident. Later on after your shift.)
4. Do you ever discuss difficult incidents with colleagues?
   a. In breaks, after work, at lunch?
   b. If so, why? If not, why not?
   c. Do you find this useful – in what way?
5. What do you think might help you to deal with situations like this in the future?
   (Prompts: Training; Supervision; Debriefing; Peer-support.)
   a. *Out of the things identified:* To what extent are these provided already?
6. Imagine you have had a particularly stressful day at work – what might you do
   after your shift had ended?
   a. Do you have a routine?
   b. How do you unwind?

    c. Do you go through the events of the day, or try to forget about them?

    d. Does this work for you?

7. Have you ever discussed work with your family or non-work colleagues?

    a. Maybe to seek advice, or to 'let off steam'?

    b. Do you find this helpful?

    c. If not, or if you do not, why is this?

The questions were designed to be open-ended, to encourage participants to explore issues and facets of EOC-related stress that were important to them individually. The interviews lasted between 40 and 70 minutes each, were audio-recorded and later transcribed for analysis. The interviews were analysed thematically, following the widely recognised method described by Braun and Clarke [27]. This approach was used as it allowed for data-driven analysis. At the time of data collection (May–July 2014), existing research on the stress experienced by dispatch personnel was limited. As such, the analytic approach needed to be primarily inductive, and allow for what Braun and Clarke refer to as 'unexpected insights'.

The participants began by explaining how their role was largely invisible to public awareness:

. . .nobody knows what we do.

(Fiona, female, 9 years in role)

Although members of the public are aware of call-handlers because they speak to them directly, and paramedics/ambulance technicians because they attend the emergency, participants stated that most people were unaware of the interim role of ambulance dispatcher. This is reflected in the scarcity of existing research concerning the role of ambulance dispatcher when compared to other EMS roles. Nick, a dispatcher with 11 years' experience in dispatch, described dispatchers as 'the faceless sort of people'. However, despite this relative invisibility, all nine participants expressed pride in the work that they did, and largely enjoyed the role:

I can honestly say I go home at the end of every single day and I've made a difference to at least one person. . . Not many people get that kind of satisfaction.

(Sam, female, 7 years in role)

The 'facelessness' of ambulance dispatch was therefore not a major concern for participants – the work is its own reward. However, the primary focus of this research was the issues of stress raised by participants. They spoke extensively about stressors, which fell into two broad categories: practical and personal. Certain practical stressors were related to wider structural issues, such as limited resources in the face of ever-increasing patient populations:

> *In dispatch, the main stressors are not having the resources, in terms of ambulances for emergencies.*

> (Jane, female, 13½ years in role)

Participants conceptualised scarcity of resources and related budgeting as unavoidable and universal issues, affecting all NHS staff. They were not overly preoccupied with them as they felt they were unchangeable at the individual, group or even regional level.

Other practical stressors were those that participants felt were inherent in the role, such as time-limited work, multi-tasking, working long shifts and exposure to trauma. Again, participants were largely accepting of these sorts of stressors, acknowledging them as fundamental features of their work and described them matter-of-factly:

> *. . .it's a maintained stress. And that's just a case of if you can take that, you'll enjoy the job.*

> (Nick, male, 11 years in role)

These practical stressors were subsequently minimised by participants until they discussed how they managed their resulting stress. The participants explained that whilst they were allotted time for breaks during their shift, staff rarely availed these. They described often working straight through their 12-hour shifts, only leaving their desks to use the toilet. Darren explained that taking a break meant removing oneself from the flow of work:

> *. . .if you took that break, you remove yourself from what is going on. In some ways it's more of a hindrance.*

> (Darren, male, 13 years in role)

As such, it was common practice for staff to choose to work through, rather than utilise breaks for rest and recovery. Paula, who had been a dispatcher for seven years, stated that the nature of the role made it 'harder to stand up, walk out and take a break', but that this was not impossible. She emphasised that breaks were available, but largely, staff actively chose not to take them. Although Darren acknowledged that this was a personal choice that contributed to his compounding stress, he also highlighted a structural failing:

> I don't think we manage our breaks well. I certainly don't. Part of that's just me, part of that's not really having the structure for that.

(Darren, male, 13 years in role)

The topic of rest and recovery was explored further by participants, particularly concerning post-shift recovery. Although participants did not describe specific routines or habits, Clive described a clear delineation between his work and personal life:

> . . .when I'm here, I'm on work time. . .When I get home, I don't want to think about it. Get it out the way.

(Clive, male, 2 years in role)

This separating of work and personal life was echoed by Jane, who suggested this type of detachment was vital for self-preservation in the role:

> . . .sometimes you have to. To protect yourself. Yeah, you do. Otherwise you'd go insane. You can't take it home with you. But it's about finding a balance.

(Jane, female, 13½ years in role)

Jane's use of the term 'finding a balance' is note-worthy considering existing literature surrounding work-related stress and the concept of allostasis. In the context of stress, allostasis refers to our ability to adapt and recover following a stressful event or situation [23, 24]. However, this is only possible if we can disengage from the stressful event after it has occurred. For Clive and Jane, this was achieved by clearly demarcating their work from their personal lives – they were able to regulate their responses following stressful work events and use their time away from work to achieve allostasis before returning to work. Conversely, Darren stated that he had no real post-shift routine and often struggled to recover from work effectively. He explained that he often returned to work the following morning feeling unrefreshed and after 13 years in the role, he no longer enjoyed his work as he once did. Having earlier explained that he struggled to manage breaks whilst on shift, Darren described how he spent considerable unstructured time after work to process:

> I went home. . . and I sat on my own there for an hour. That's an hour – gone. Just to unwind.

(Darren, male, 13 years in role)

Likely, Darren was not truly 'unwinding' from work, but passively ruminating on stressful events from his shift [28]. Even when 'off the clock', it is likely that Darren was still psychologically 'at work', leaving him in a state of heightened arousal (i.e. stressed). Not being able to sufficiently recover, workers like Darren return to their next shift already feeling stressed – this can have a cumulative effect (referred to as allostatic load) and can potentially deplete our tolerance for otherwise manageable stressful events. The work itself was not necessarily any more stressful than before, but Darren's insufficient recovery strategies left him less able to cope. The role itself involves periods of acute stress, but when insufficiently managed can lead to chronic stress in staff, risking burnout [29–31]. Work-related burnout is a state of psychological, emotional and even physical exhaustion, caused by prolonged stress and feeling overwhelmed. It is characterised by feelings of helplessness and increasing cynicism, disengagement or loss of motivation in work, depersonalisation and compassion fatigue. It can contribute to ongoing mental and physical ill-health, as well as affecting work-engagement and productivity. Not only are healthcare workers at a high risk of burnout but the impacts this may have on their ongoing work are cause for serious concern.

Some participants clearly managed their work stressors better than others, demonstrated by the length of time they remained in the role, and the positive way they spoke about their work experiences. However, their difficulty in identifying specific coping mechanisms, and in the case of Darren having any strategies for stress-management at all, highlights the importance of structured support systems. Darren is by no means an isolated case – healthcare research and survey data demonstrate that healthcare workers are particularly at risk of allostatic load, emotional exhaustion and burnout [32–35]. To address this, supporting staff to develop adequate recovery and coping strategies is of paramount importance.

The personal stressors participants described were predominantly interpersonal issues with other staff groups, such as how their role was often compared to that of frontline EMS staff:

> *Your role in control is not seen as particularly attractive. . . like you're a necessity but you're enabling what's really important.*

> (Sam, female, 7 years in role)

This was reflected in the implicit attitudes of Terry, a dispatcher with six years' experience in dispatch, who saw working in the EOC as simply 'a stepping stone' to become a paramedic. These perceptions echo findings from existing research concerning police dispatchers in the United States [22]. All nine participants highlighted this as a significant source of stress. Participants felt as though the importance of their role was overlooked or actively minimised by other members of staff. Worse still, Nick explained that dispatch staff often felt maltreated by paramedic staff:

> *. . .everyone says we're like a buffer. . . the crews, who are they gonna talk to? That's no excuse. If I have stress, I don't get, I'm not snapping at a crew am I?*

And barking orders at them because I'm upset about something. It doesn't work like that.

(Nick, male, 11 years in role)

Participants such as Sam and Nick described the personal efforts they made to forge positive working relationships with their paramedic colleagues. Nick described treating everyone with 'respect and a bit of courtesy', emphasising that one could 'do the job professionally but. . . still be kind to people'.

The only apparent structural arrangement to encourage inter-team understanding was that dispatch staff were allowed (and encouraged) to shadow two paramedic shifts per year. Conversely, paramedics were not actively encouraged to undertake similar shadowing in the EOC. Paramedics visited the EOC during their orientation in initial training. Participants explained that subsequently, paramedics only ever shadowed EOC work if a complaint about their conduct to EOC staff had been raised. They speculated that this was seen as a punishment rather than an opportunity for mutual understanding or relationship development.

Sam took this further, sacrificing personal time to work directly with paramedic staff. She explained this helped forge meaningful relationships with staff and made her work 'far easier'. However, she posed the poignant question, 'as a dispatcher, why is that your responsibility?' Participants highlighted that there were no formal structures in place to support this type of interpersonal development and as such, limited mutual understanding of others' roles.

Paramedics are directly exposed to patient trauma and distress. This may contribute to compassion fatigue and depersonalisation [29, 36] of dispatch staff, with whom they primarily liaised with remotely. Ron, who fulfilled a dual-role as a dispatcher and part-time emergency medical technician, was able to provide insights from both sides. He emphasised a need for mutual understanding in forging positive working relationships:

. . .you'd see so many crews that would get so frustrated, stuff happening, things come up on screen, go here do that, and they didn't know why. . . as you know I have a background in the dispatch centre, even just spending 12 hours with someone in an ambulance, you can say to them "oh this is why they're doing that". . . suddenly it all makes sense.

(Ron, male, 15 years in role)

These accounts highlighted participants' perceived burden of effort – they recognised the importance of and need for good working relationships with colleagues on the frontline, but this was not reflected in formal training and team structure. Participants felt personal pressure to create these working relationships outside of their structured work time. By taking an active role in forging a better wider-team working environment, Nick, Ron and Sam demonstrated an awareness of the 'bigger picture', beyond the workings of the EOC. Although dispatch staff were a physically separate team, being able to work effectively with frontline staff was vital to the smooth running of EMS.

Although participants made no overt complaints about supervisory support, they did allude to this as an area needing more attention. There was limited mention of supervision or line management support, as this was rarely available or offered. Instead, participants described an atmosphere of implicit peer support, with all staff 'in it together'.

Most participants discussed staff training as a potential supportive mechanism. Jane explained that appropriate training could not only help staff feel prepared and more confident, it also helped them feel valued and supported:

> . . .you're investing in them. They feel cared about. They think, oh you're taking care of me, I've got what I need, I've got everything I need, I've got the full package. I'm a professional.

> (Jane, female, 13½ years in role)

Several participants highlighted training as a missed opportunity. Participants explained that training days were often multidisciplinary so, in theory, an opportunity for structured team building. However, Darren explained that whilst they did receive regular training, he felt it was 'a bit lacking' and not always relevant to all staff involved. It is possible, if not even likely, that those staff who felt a training session was irrelevant to them resented attending, or that their valuable time was being ill-spent.

FUTURE DIRECTIONS

As with any qualitative research endeavour, this study reflects the phenomenological experiences of a limited participant group. Although participants were purposefully recruited to represent a breadth of ages, years' experience in the role and varying personal experiences, the views expressed by participants may not be reflective of dispatch staff working in different NHS Trusts. However, given these findings corroborate existing research into EMS staff experiences of stress, it is likely they are translatable to other settings.

The participants in this research described how they found their role rewarding and took pride in the work they did. This reflects the wider picture of staff in caring roles, concerning work motivation and meaningful work. Participants conceptualised certain extra-person stressors, such as limited resources and long shifts without taking breaks (although these were allotted), as simply 'part of the job'. One participant expressed that if one could endure these extreme stressors, the role was enjoyable. Whether the participants found the role rewarding was not under question, given the core of staff who had been in the role for 10 years or more. This intrinsic motivation and benefit-finding likely act as meaningful coping strategies in the face of overtly stressful work. However, by normalising certain modes of working, staff risk perpetuating a culture which accepts a high rate of burnout as part of the job description.

The participants in this study described several changes they had made to positively affect their working environment. These included active efforts to improve interpersonal relationships with paramedic staff. As identified by García-Izquierdo and Ríos-Rísquez [35], interpersonal conflict is a significant predicting factor in burnout amongst EMS staff. Whilst seemingly simple, by making personal efforts to develop good relationships with outside-team members, participants were able to have positive interactions with them going forwards and reduce the frequency of unresolved interpersonal conflict [37]. This could potentially reduce the amount of 'deferred stress', when (as described by Nick) paramedics use dispatch staff as a buffer for their own work-related stress. Shared, mutual understanding of roles can also positively change how different teams perceive each other's roles, helping to address dispatchers' feelings of facelessness or invisibility compared to frontline EMS staff.

The issue then is where the responsibility for this interpersonal bonding lies. Participants explained that whilst they were allowed and encouraged to take two shifts per year 'on the road' with paramedic crews, this was difficult to arrange owing to ongoing staff shortages. Participants explained that interpersonal relationship work was often undertaken in their otherwise free-time and was not actively structured in their role development or training. For those unwilling or unable to give the time, the issue of interpersonal conflict persisted. For those who chose to sacrifice personal time, there was a trade-off between this and improved working relationships. For this latter group, there is the potential for blurred work-leisure boundaries, and this introduces a risk of insufficient out-of-work recovery and burnout later.

Rather than relying on the initiative or willingness of individual staff members, team-building could be integrated with existing training and support provisions. This could include regular cross-team shadowing, with a focus on developing working relationships and mutual understanding. It might also involve re-structuring multi-disciplinary training events, with an explicit focus on positive and effective communication, skills sharing and mental well-being. Not only will this communicate to staff the importance of wider-team working but it also has the potential to improve morale and boost productivity [38–40].

Team training is also an open opportunity to identify and implement structured support for those staff members who may be showing early signs of chronic stress and potential burnout. Jane, Nick, Ron and Darren had similar levels of experience in role (11–15 years), but unlike his colleagues, Darren stated that he no longer found his work as enjoyable or fulfilling as he once had. This was likely due in part to his inability to effectively recover from work-related stress off shift. Well-being interventions and psychoeducation is potentially relevant to all EMS staff groups and can have long-term benefits for workers whose jobs are inherently stressful [17, 41, 42]. Given the vital nature of the work coupled with an ongoing high rate of staff turnover in the

NHS [43], developing effective strategies for supporting staff mental well-being and coping is of paramount importance. Future research should explore specific trends in stress-coping and staff attrition, and the potential efficacy of structured support interventions.

REFERENCES

1. Galeano, R. (2019). Understanding the health of operational personnel in an ambulance service: a mixed methods study. PhD thesis. Queensland University of Technology.
2. Gardett, I., Trefts, E., Olola, C., and Scott, G. (2020). Unique job roles and mental health risk factors among emergency dispatchers. In: *Mental Health Intervention and Treatment of First Responders and Emergency Workers*, 49–62. Hershey, PA: IGI Global.
3. Golding, S.E., Horsfield, C., Davies, A. et al. (2017). Exploring the psychological health of emergency dispatch centre operatives: a systematic review and narrative synthesis. *PeerJ* 5: e3735.
4. Office for National Statistics (2019). Sickness absence in the labour market: 2018.
5. Office for National Statistics (2018). Sickness absence falls to the lowest rate on record – Office for National Statistics [Internet]. www.ons.gov.uk/employmentandlabourmarket/peopleinwork/employmentandemployeetypes/articles/sicknessabsencefallstothelowestratein24years/2018-07-30 (accessed 3 December 2019).
6. The King's Fund (2019). NHS sickness absence: let's talk about mental health [Internet]. www.kingsfund.org.uk/blog/2019/10/nhs-sickness-absence (accessed 6 December 2019).
7. UNISON (2014). Stress epidemic stretches ambulance service to breaking point [Internet]. www.unison.org.uk/news/stress-epidemic-stretches-ambulance-service-to-breaking-point (accessed 13 December 2014).
8. Khamisa, N., Oldenburg, B., Peltzer, K., and Ilic, D. (2015). Work related stress, burnout, job satisfaction and general health of nurses. *International Journal of Environmental Research and Public Health* 12 (1): 652–666.
9. Adali, E., Priami, M., Evagelou, H. et al. (2003). Burnout in psychiatric nursing personnel in Greek hospitals. *European Journal of Psychiatry* 17 (3): 173–181.
10. Tuvesson, H., Eklund, M., and Wann-Hansson, C. (2011). Perceived stress among nursing staff in psychiatric inpatient care: the influence of perceptions of the ward atmosphere and the psychosocial work environment. *Issues in Mental Health Nursing* 32 (7): 441–448.
11. Thompson, C.V., Naumann, D.N., Fellows, J.L. et al. (2017). Post-traumatic stress disorder amongst surgical trainees: an unrecognised risk? *The Surgeon* 15 (3): 123–130.
12. Anton, N.E., Montero, P.N., Howley, L.D. et al. (2015). What stress coping strategies are surgeons relying upon during surgery? In: *American Journal of Surgery*, 846–851. Elsevier.

13. Dimou, F.M., Eckelbarger, D., and Riall, T.S. (2016). Surgeon burnout: a systematic review. *Journal of the American College of Surgeons* 222 (6): 1230–1239.

14. Adriaenssens, J., de Gucht, V., and Maes, S. (2012). The impact of traumatic events on emergency room nurses: findings from a questionnaire survey. *International Journal of Nursing Studies* 49 (11): 1411–1422.

15. Leblanc, V.R., Regehr, C., Tavares, W. et al. (2012). The impact of stress on paramedic performance during simulated critical events. *Prehospital and Disaster Medicine* 27 (4): 369–374.

16. Wankhade, P. (2016). Staff perceptions and changing role of pre-hospital profession in the UK ambulance services: an exploratory study. *International Journal of Emergency Services* 5 (2): 126–144.

17. Austin, C.L., Pathak, M., and Thompson, S. (2018). Secondary traumatic stress and resilience among EMS. *Journal of Paramedic Practice* 10 (6): 240–247.

18. Farquharson, B., Allan, J., Johnston, D. et al. (2012). Stress amongst nurses working in a healthcare telephone-advice service: relationship with job satisfaction, intention to leave, sickness absence, and performance. *Journal of Advanced Nursing* 68 (7): 1624–1635.

19. Allan, J.L., Farquharson, B., Choudhary, C.J. et al. (2014). Stress in telephone helpline nurses is associated with failures of concentration, attention and memory, and with more conservative referral decisions. *Journal of Advanced Nursing* 105 (2): 200–213.

20. Adams, K., Shakespeare-Finch, J., and Armstrong, D. (2015). An interpretative phenomenological analysis of stress and well-being in emergency medical dispatchers. *Journal of Loss and Trauma* 20 (5): 430–448.

21. Gurevich, M., Halpern, J., Brazeau, P. et al. (2009). *Frontline Stress behind the Scenes: Emergency Medical Dispatchers*. Toronto, ON: Association of Public Safety Communications Officials.

22. Burke, T.W. (1999). Dispatcher stress. In: *Protect Your Life!: A Health Handbook for Law Enforcement Professionals* (ed. D.C. Umeh), 79–86. Looseleaf Law Publication.

23. Payne, R. and Fletcher, B. (1980). Stress and work: a review and theoretical framework, I. *Personnel Review* 9: 19–29.

24. Payne, R. and Fletcher, B. (1980). Stress at work: a review and theoretical framework, II. *Personnel Review* 9: 5–8.

25. Forslund, K., Kihlgren, a., and Kihlgren, M. (2004). Operators' experiences of emergency calls. *Journal of Telemedicine and Telecare* [Internet] 10 (5): 290–297. http://jtt.sagepub.com/lookup/doi/10.1258/1357633042026323 (accessed 29 March 2014).

26. Coxon, A., Cropley, M., Schofield, P. et al. (2016). 'You're never making just one decision': exploring the lived experiences of ambulance Emergency Operations Centre personnel. *Emergency Medicine Journal* 33 (9): 645–651.

27. Braun, V. and Clarke, V. (2006). Using thematic analysis in psychology. *Qualitative Research in Psychology* 3 (2): 77–101.

28. Querstret, D. and Cropley, M. (2012). Exploring the relationship between work-related rumination, sleep quality and work-related fatigue. *Journal of Occupational Health Psychology* 17 (3): 341–353.

29. Weibel, L., Gabrion, I., Aussedat, M., and Kreutz, G. (2003). Work-related stress in an emergency medical dispatch center. *Annals of Emergency Medicine* 41 (4): 500–506.

30. Maslach, C. and Jackson, S.E. (1981). The measurement of experienced burnout. *Journal of Organizational Behavior* 2: 99–113.

31. Maslach, C. and Leiter, M.P. (2008). Early predictors of job burnout and engagement. *The Journal of Applied Psychology* 93: 498–512.

32. Rössler, W. (2012). Stress, burnout, and job dissatisfaction in mental health workers. *European Archives of Psychiatry and Clinical Neuroscience* 262: 65–69.

33. Jonsson, A. and Segesten, K. (2004). Guilt, shame and need for a container: a study of post-traumatic stress among ambulance personnel. *Accident and Emergency Nursing* 12 (4): 215–223.

34. Gokcen, C., Zengin, S., Oktay, M. et al. (2013). Burnout, job satisfaction and depression in the healthcare personnel who work in the emergency department. *Anatolian Journal of Psychiatry* 14: 122–128.

35. García-Izquierdo, M. and Ríos-Rísquez, M.I. (2012). The relationship between psychosocial job stress and burnout in emergency departments: an exploratory study. *Nursing Outlook* 60 (5): 322–329.

36. Halpern, J., Maunder, R.G., Schwartz, B., and Gurevich, M. (2012). Identifying, describing, and expressing emotions after critical incidents in paramedics. *Journal of Traumatic Stress* 25 (1): 111–114.

37. Apker, J., Propp, K.M., Zabava Ford, W.S., and Hofmeister, N. (2006). Collaboration, credibility, compassion, and coordination: professional nurse communication skill sets in health care team interactions. *Journal of Professional Nursing* 22 (3): 180–189.

38. Klein, C., DiazGranados, D., Salas, E. et al. (2009). Does team building work? *Small Group Research* 40: 181–222.

39. Salas, E., Rozell, D., Mullen, B., and Driskell, J.E. (1999). The effect of team building on performance: an integration. *Small Group Research* 30: 309–329.

40. Tannenbaum, S.I., Beard, R.L., and Salas, E. (1992). Chapter 5 Team building and its influence on team effectiveness: an examination of conceptual and empirical developments. *Advances in Psychology* 82: 117–153.

41. Lawn, S.J., Willis, E.M., Roberts, L., et al. (2019). Ambulance Employees Association – Scoping literature reviews drawing on qualitative literature to address the physical, psychological, psychobiological, and psychosocial health of operational ambulance staff and interventions to address the impact of workplace stressors. https://dspace2.flinders.edu.au/xmlui/handle/2328/39227 (accessed 3 December 2019).

42. Anshel, M.H., Umscheid, D., and Brinthaupt, T.M. (2012). Effect of a combined coping skills and wellness program on perceived stress and physical energy among police emergency dispatchers: an exploratory study. *Journal of Police and Criminal Psychology* 28 (1): 1–14.

43. Buchan, J., Charlesworth, A., Gerschlick, B., and Seccombe, I. (2019). A critical moment: NHS staffing trends, retention and attrition [Internet]. London. www.health.org.uk/sites/default/files/upload/publications/2019/A Critical Moment_1.pdf (accessed 17 December 2019).

CHAPTER 5

Paramedics' Lived Experiences of Post-Incident Traumatic Distress and Psychosocial Support

An Interpretative Phenomenological Study

Joanne Mildenhall

Faculty of Health & Applied Sciences, University of the West of England, Bristol, UK

The realities of clinical practice for paramedics and ambulance personnel expose emotional and social complexities which are often ambiguous and shared within an environment that is often unpredictable. Whilst the ebb and flow of the work may be perceived as routine and perhaps even mundane, there is a reality that one never knows quite what will happen or be faced with when on shift. At times, ambulance personnel may be presented with highly distressing cases of human suffering, social deprivation and isolation, illness and injury; occasionally on a catastrophic scale. They often face incidents as a crew of two or three (usually configured as a paramedic, a less clinically trained or unqualified member of staff and a student paramedic) or as a solo responder. Thus, there is a real pressure of responsibility associated with providing clinical care in often challenging situations. This is particularly the case where the working environment presents physical and psychological risks, including threats to personal safety from violence when attending emergency calls [1–3]. Sadly, despite new legislation to protect ambulance staff [4], reports indicate that incidents of abuse have continued [5, 6].

Much has been written on the psychological complexities of trauma exposure within emergency responder populations, with a seemingly general consensus that for this particular occupational group, it is incidents which provoke subjective feelings of

The Mental Health and Wellbeing of Healthcare Practitioners: Research and Practice, First Edition.
Edited by Esther Murray and Jo Brown.
© 2021 John Wiley & Sons Ltd. Published 2021 by John Wiley & Sons Ltd.

being emotionally overwhelmed; for example, where personnel have developed an emotional connection with those whom they are caring for [7] or through experiencing death or serious injury to another; particularly in the case of paediatric patients, family, friends or colleagues. Experiencing trauma-related distress in these circumstances is in keeping with the Diagnostic and Statistical Manual of Mental Disorders (DSM-5) definition of trauma as 'the exposure to actual or threatened death, serious injury or sexual violation' witnessed through personal experience as it occurs to other people, learning that the event occurred to someone in their family or a close friend, or 'through repeated or extreme exposure to adverse details of the event' [8] which 'applies to workers who encounter the consequences of traumatic events as part of their professional responsibilities' [9].

Mishra et al. [7] noted that of a sample of 101 Emergency Medical Service personnel in Hawaii (45% response rate), 88% disclosed having experienced personal psychological distress following incidents they had attended at work. Distressing situations included serious injury or death of a co-worker, infant death, paediatric trauma and caring for upset relatives. More recent studies have identified that these healthcare workers are regularly exposed to incidents with elements of trauma; either vicariously or through direct observation from being on the scene and witnessing the aftermath of injury or illness [2, 10, 11]. Thus, not only is the psychological impact of a single traumatic incident of real concern, but also the chronic, accumulative exposure to distressing events which poses a considerable threat to a responder's psychological wellbeing. As such, it is now recognised that this clinical cohort of frontline workers are at risk of psycho-emotional distress/overload, post-traumatic symptomology and/or moral injury [7, 12–14].

Critically, previous studies have emphasised post-incident psychopathological outcomes including anxiety, depression and acute stress, with research focused upon clinical interventions such as cognitive-behavioural therapy. However, there has been less sociological inquiry into cultural discourses and the symbolic language associated with mental distress of emergency practitioners working within the ambulance sector.

From the limited studies available, we know that embodied within the occupational and professional culture of these workers is a discourse which is ambiguous in terms of attitudes towards workplace stress and post-incident recovery. The discourse draws upon linguistic metaphors which *minimise* distress and thus make it significantly challenging for individuals to engage in any display of emotion or seek help for their psycho-emotional health due to fear of perceived stigma from others, perceived negative impact upon career progression and heightened anxiety at the prospect of being referred to registering bodies regarding their fitness to practice [15, 16]. As noted, published research is scant, particularly within United Kingdom emergency responder populations. Furthermore, relatively few studies have been undertaken within the workplace sector to examine in depth the efficacy of resilience-enhancing factors which could be key to understanding positive growth and emotional adjustment following trauma exposure. Such studies will be fundamental to developing our knowledge of psychological wellbeing, particularly in the face of adversity [17].

One factor renowned for mediating distress is that of positively experienced social support. Trauma psychologists have theorised that feeling supported and talking through our experiences enables the integration and processing of trauma memories from the brain's thalamo-amygdala memory pathway to the psycho-neurological hippocampal pathway which has been determined as key to processing experiences from short-term into long-term memory [18]. This is believed to be vital in mediating the impact of traumatic distress responses (such as intrusive memories) within individuals.

From a psychosocial perspective, the basic human need to connect with and talk through distressing experiences often provides comfort and reassurance for affected individuals, promotes feelings of belonging, cohesion and acceptance and potentially alleviates any feelings of isolation [19, 20]. In addition, it is hypothesised that when an individual is ready to, retelling the narrative of an incident has the effect of lessening overwhelming emotions and enables shared sense-making of the event to occur. This is particularly important to emergency personnel who frequently recount narratives of incidents within their peer group [21, 22]. However, this is often undertaken on a professional and practical level (detailing the medical condition, challenges, skills used and treatments) rather than engaging in any personal emotional reflexion. Certainly, within published research, there is little exploring the ambiguous emotional complexities associated with the occupational culture and work of ambulance personnel, and limited in-depth study of their lived experiences. There appears to be negligible engagement with the voice of these frontline workers or their personal experiences of support following a distressing call.

The current study, therefore, through phenomenological inquiry, gathered rich dialogic and narrative data to explore the life-world experiences of National Health Service (NHS) ambulance personnel who felt that they had, through the course of their work, been exposed to at least one incident that was psychologically distressing to them. To reduce the risk of memory bias, the incident was to have occurred no longer than five years previously.

Ethical approval was granted by the University of Nottingham and the host NHS Ambulance Service prior to participant recruitment. Six participants employed by one NHS ambulance service in England were engaged with the study. To maintain anonymity, all were allocated pseudonyms, only known to the principle researcher.

In terms of demographics, there was an equal split of males/females within the cohort. They had variable lengths of service from just over a year, to more than 20 years. Two of the participants were ambulance technicians, two were paramedics, one was an ambulance nurse and the other was a team leader (first-line manager). Only one participant had a regular crewmate. The remainder of the sample either worked alone or with a variety of colleagues.

Face-to-face semi-structured interviews were undertaken to explore the phenomenon in question. This data collection method also allowed for flexibility in that participants were free to tell their narrative experiences with their own meanings, beliefs and assumptions. The aim was to seek privileged insight into their world, to 'see' their experiences through their eyes and to gain an understanding of what it was really like to be that frontline healthcare clinician attending scenes of distress, and of their experiences of post-incident psychosocial support.

Interviews were conducted by the author and continued until they seemed to reach a natural end and no new data emerged (as agreed by both the participant and the researcher). On average, the interviews lasted for one hour. The questions explored the participants' personal distress associated with the incident, their psycho-emotional and behavioural responses to that particular call, the coping mechanisms they drew upon if any and their experiences of support post-incident.

All interviews were tape-recorded and transcribed verbatim. Coding of the transcripts was undertaken and cross-checked with the participants. Interpretative phenomenological analysis was used to identify themes from the data. Systematic iterative examination and thematic analysis initially revealed many categories which were subsequently reduced to key themes and sub themes. Given the succinctness of this chapter, the main themes will only be discussed briefly.

DISTRESS

In talking of their occupational trauma exposure, all participants described experiencing varying levels of psychological distress either prior to, during or in the immediate post-incident phase, until the research interview date, which for some of the participants was only a few months later, whilst for others was a couple of years later.

Rebecca, a newly qualified graduate paramedic, talked of being en route to her first paediatric cardiac arrest. She described how her anxiety and apprehension grew as they drew nearer to the scene:

> *I just remember sitting there [in the ambulance] on the way, and just um, I remember holding on to the inside of the door handle and I could feel my hand getting really, really sweaty. . . I didn't know what I was gonna find and I think it was partly that fear of the unknown. . .*

> [p. 5]

Following the call, Rebecca explained the emotional distress she felt in the days after the call:

> *. . .at the time, I really felt like I was suppressing my emotions, um, I was really suppressing them, pushing them down. . . .*

> [p. 12]

Through exploring this further with her, Rebecca indicated that her use of suppression was an attempt to control the overwhelming emotions that she was feeling, to enable her to function and continue working as a paramedic. In doing so, she had attempted to hide her emotions from colleagues, and to a degree, from her conscious self. Whilst this may be a coping strategy in the short-term enabling her to perform her professional role, by suppressing (and avoiding) emotions, in the longer-term, it is more likely that an individual will have difficulty processing memories of the event and thus develop an extended post-traumatic response [23]. Indeed, in Lowery and Stokes' [16] quantitative study of seventy-four student paramedics who were training within an Australian Ambulance Service, there was found to be a correlative link between attitudes towards emotional expression and exacerbated traumatic reactions.

Richard, an ex-military, highly experienced and long-standing paramedic, expressed great difficulty following his attendance at a different paediatric arrest, whereby at the scene, the child was deemed to be beyond resuscitation. He said, that for months afterwards:

> *I was getting flashbacks. I was getting an hours' sleep a night. I was. . . going to bed. . . and getting up after an hour; couldn't sleep. So, I'd be pacing around the house and I'd be sitting there. . . I replayed every second of that job in my head thinking 'could I have done anything different?'. I could've very easily at a couple of points, could've. . . topped myself, because. . . I've never been so low in my life.*

[p. 7/8]

Each participant discussed how the experiences of attending their particular call had a long-lasting psychological impact. Richard found it very difficult to cope with the recurrent intrusive memories, dreams and ruminating thoughts which he described as being intensely felt. His response was prolonged, and his level of distress impacted upon his life such that he required time away from work. Symbolically through his use of language it was noticeable that Richard disclosed that his avoidance of work was not only due to psychological incapacity but was also representative of a means of avoiding overwhelming thoughts and feelings associated with the incident. For him, the workplace served as reminder of the event and at the time of the interview, approximately eighteen months later, Richard still held significant negative beliefs towards those whom he felt represented the organisation and whom he felt had betrayed his loyal and long service, in not providing him with post-incident psychological safety and support. Explicit within his language, Richard divulged feelings of rejection by his employer which appeared to translate into feeling alienated, isolated, and feeling victimised.

At the time of the incident and for months afterwards, he shared how he had turned to alcohol and medications to help numb his distress in an effort to help him cope. Arguably, this use of maladaptive coping strategies was also in some way, his attempt to regulate his fluctuating and distressing emotions, which were felt as extremely painful. Yet, his desire to avoid and suppress this pain hampered his ability to regulate his emotions by other means, as is often the case in those who experience post-traumatic stress [24].

George, a Team Leader who had been employed in the Service for some years, had attended the cardiac arrest of a close family member. He shared how, in the months afterwards, he felt 'unusually' and 'randomly' upset and angry with what he perceived had 'no apparent trigger'. In the immediate aftermath, he explained:

> *I can't really describe how I felt, but it was probably every single emotion that was available. Just felt let down, disappointed, angry, upset, stressed, just every-thing. Just felt this overwhelming kind of um surge of emotion and just kind of walked out and felt that basically, I had to punch the first thing I could find really, which was the side of the [ambulance] vehicle um and went 'round the corner and just sort of placed my thoughts really.. . .'*

[p. 5]

Vix, an experienced ambulance technician, recounted her narrative of attending the emergency call to resuscitate her new-born God-daughter. Sadly, the little girl was unable to be saved despite every effort of Vix, her crew and the hospital paediatric team. Whilst knowing that she had provided the best clinical care she and the team could, Vix intimately shared how she had experienced overwhelming guilt and shame which appeared to remain with her to the day of the research interview (three years later). She said:

> *I don't know why it still bothers me but still. . . . so you know, no-one blames. . . blames me or us as a crew. . . but I don't know, I still feel guilty about it.. . .*

[p. 7]

Her voice trailed off and for a moment, she appeared deep in thought, somewhat dissociated and appearing to be recalling that moment again. It seemed that she had been released from any blame by her friend but held herself critically to account for the loss of the baby's life, for which she continued to feel deep, immeasurable, distressing guilt and although not specifically named by her, it was apparent that she experienced intrapersonal trauma and deeply internalised shame, altering her core beliefs about herself from that of a 'good' person, to someone who had developed negative self-perceptions. Indeed, Scoglio et al. [24] noted that 'shame following traumatic experiences can have a profound and pervasive effect on personal identity. The self may be seen as defective, inherently bad, deserving of maltreatment, and something that must be kept hidden from others' [p. 2018]. Arguably, shame extends to professional identity also, and may be associated with emotional detachment, withdrawal and exhaustion [25].

AMBIVALENCE OF TALKING

Analysis of the participants' narratives revealed conflicting differences in beliefs and attitudes towards openly talking about how they felt after the incident. In terms of a reluctance to talk, various themes emerged from the participants' narratives. This included a sense of risk around sharing one's feelings, particularly in terms of the perceived impact upon reputation and threats to one's identity and/or gender:

> *I think there is a little bit of a stigma..if you..say you're not coping..it's a little bit of a sign of weakness, especially as a woman; 'ooh yeah [laughs] bloody women, going home all stressed, can't cope with the job [said sarcastically] but you just have to talk about it and admit that you're not coping and I think. . . ask for help.*

> Vix [p. 15]

> *What I wish had happened that day was that I um. . . that I would have gone home and cried for the rest of the day. . . but I, I just know that I wouldn't ever have wanted the others to think that I was weak. . .*

> Rebecca [p. 17]

Asked if she felt her colleagues would have considered her weak if she had cried, Rebecca answered with no time for thought; 'yes, I do' and placed considerable emphasis on her female gender as being the confounding factor. She anticipated that fellow staff may have viewed her as:

> *. . .Just some kind of hysterical woman.. . .*

> [p. 12]

> *. . .I don't like to think of the male members of staff like, thinking of me as weak. . . I want them to think I'm a good paramedic; that I'm a strong person. . . that's what I see as good qualities.. . .*

> [p. 19]

Here, Rebecca gave insight into the fundamental assumptions and cultural beliefs that she held regarding professional identity of what makes a 'good' paramedic. There appeared to be incongruence between her state of being (particularly challenging her gendered notion of being female) and positioning herself within a perceived 'macho' culture. This seemed to represent a real dichotomous pressure for both Vix and Rebecca who sought to transgress the cultural norms and rules associated with emotional display by refraining from revealing their emotions and from seeking support so that they avoided the shame of appearing vulnerable or weak in front of their colleagues, thereby maintaining their concept of professional identity as 'good' ambulance clinicians, and perhaps, importantly to them at the time, they reduced a fear of being judged, or from becoming disconnected from their professional social group, their colleagues. However, arguably, without being able to share their feelings and emotions, both females were left experiencing considerable internalised distress.

The consequences of not talking (through personal choice, perceived stigma or due to other factors) were noted. Vix disclosed that from her experience:

> *You know, it's easier just to bury it, keep pushing it down and avoiding any situation where you have to deal with it or talk about it, you know, it's easier to carry on with your life, and then, it pops up.. . .*

[p. 15]

Despite the perceptions of risk around talking, or more so, in sharing one's emotions and feelings, all participants highly valued talking as a coping strategy. Indeed, when asked what their advice would be to others, all said 'talk, talk and talk'. They suggested that talking to those crewmates and colleagues who were trusted, was in fact helpful to their psychological wellbeing, particularly in enabling them to process and assimilate the event with those who held a shared professional understanding and connected humanity in terms of providing empathy. Talking essentially provided an emotional outlet and helped to 'put things into perspective'. In a state of apparent post-incident emotional hyperarousal, this informal psychosocial care appeared to be of comfort to the participants, influencing emotional regulation and providing the psychological safety of feeling socially connected and emotionally contained within their close occupational community:

> *Everyone was a bit subdued, but we had a cup of tea and just chatted about it, and I think we all knew that we need to talk to each other a bit more.. . .*

Archie [p. 5]

Richard also highlighted his perception of the longer-term impact of not talking about traumatic experiences. He positioned talking as a preventative measure and resilience factor essential for ambulance work:

> *. . .because otherwise we're gonna have such a burn out rate. . . and I think that we're gonna be paying the price for that.. . .*

[p. 7]

INFORMAL AND FORMAL SUPPORT AT WORK

In particular, most of the participants felt that it was extremely helpful to talk with crewmates, the colleague(s) whom they had experienced the incident alongside.

I think it's nice in a way, to have, to be able to talk to somebody, somebody else who's going through the same situation.. . . .

Vix [p. 15]

Mary, who attended a fatal motorcycle collision, added:

It was good [to keep working with him]..because we bounced off each other and as to whether everything was normal..whether, you know, if you were still dealing with it, and obviously [telling someone] if they weren't there, they wouldn't have experienced it, or telling somebody about what it's like. . . is totally different.

[p. 14]

Mary highlighted the importance of sharing emotional responses with the colleague who had attended the incident with her. Through the bonded connection that they had with each other, they were able to normalise how they felt; a process that she believed would have been more challenging, with someone who had not experienced the incident in the role as a medic.

In terms of their employing organisation, the participants' narratives revealed an inconsistency in their experiences of post-incident support from managers. Some of the participants found their managers wholly supportive following the incident, whereas for others, they found it to be lacking. However, all interviewees noted how important a source of support managers and team leaders were or could be, both on a personal level and in providing guidance and access to other formal support processes.

For example, Archie, who attended a particularly horrific murder of a young female, said that immediately after the call:

The um, um Bronze. . . err.. . . declined to come and see us, so we talked to each other about what had happened (sounds sad). . . they didn't think it was serious enough.. . . .

[p. 5]

Bronze not coming in was, or no one sort of bothering from the management side of things was like um. . . it wasn't um, um so much as 'Oh my, no one's bothered', it was kind of like 'that's what we expected. . . that's what's expected.. . . .

[p. 6]

To have the post-incident support of the Bronze Officer (an operational manager) was important to Archie. However, he alluded within his narrative that this was not forthcoming and had not been experienced on previous occasions. This was a general consensus amongst the participants who felt that a lack of compassionate understanding towards psychological distress from their leadership team was a significant influencing factor upon their recovery from the event:

> *I think I felt quite let down and very devalued at that point. . . I just felt that a little bit more understanding would have gone a long way.. . .*

> George [p. 8]

On the contrary, Vix stated:

> *I spoke to my team leader, and they were brilliant.*

> [p. 10]

Formal supports also included counselling and post-incident defusing (referred to in-house as debriefing). Again, some ambivalence was noted, with scepticism and fear of emotional exposure being of concern. However, once the participants had worked through any internal conflict and sought therapeutic assistance, the majority found it to be a positive and enhancing experience, helping to process the incident.

> *I found them to be really good. Yeah, I was quite pleased with it really.*

> George [p. 6]

SUPPORT OUTSIDE OF WORK

Outside of work, the participants expressed the need for a close relationship with someone with whom they could 'off-load' to. It was important that there was someone who could listen and hear what they needed to say, who could understand the impact of the incident upon them and who also had the capacity to hold and contain the paramedic's narrative and emotional experiences. However, in contrast to this, there remained a personal need to protect close family and friends from vicarious traumatisation, thereby shielding them from hearing about the horrors and images that were experienced, because of an appreciation that this may have caused distress to them.

> *I don't feel that I should burden them with things like that, urm, you know, it's not their choice that I do this job and see horrible things.. . .*

> Rebecca [p. 24]

Discussion

This interpretative phenomenological study intended to explore ambulance personnel's experiences of emotional distress following attendance at a traumatic emergency call, and of post-incident psychosocial support.

All participants experienced both somatic and psychological distress following attendance at their respective calls, and self-reported that their symptomology had continued for a considerable time following the event (for most participants, this was over one year). Reactions varied from physical symptoms such as unusual recurrent minor illnesses and fatigue to psychological effects including intrusive re-experiencing of memories in the form of nightmares and flashbacks. This finding is concurrent with that of many other studies engaging emergency services workers [2, 26, 27]. These outcomes, however, must be held in balance as other studies report that whilst paramedics may develop post-incident sequelae, there is also evidence to suggest that many ambulance employees positively reframe traumatic experiences in terms of clinical and professional practice outcomes (such as using clinical knowledge and skills to provide quality care, collaborative team-working) which is felt as challenging yet rewarding and satisfying [28]. This may contribute towards post-traumatic growth.

In terms of post-incident support, the rich dialogic data provided by the participants, uncovered emotional dissonance with internal conflict between one's authentic emotions and beliefs, with an uneasiness around acknowledging and showing emotional vulnerability with colleagues and significant others, such as managers. Inextricably linked was a fear of emotional exposure threatening their professional identity and anxiety surrounding cultural stigma and how they may be perceived if they displayed how they truly felt. This was particularly illustrated within the narratives of Vix and Rebecca, who through their disclosures also highlighted the presence of gendered discourses towards mental health and emotional display within their occupational culture. Independently, these female participants talked of feeling unease at revealing their true emotions associated with the incidents they had attended due to their perception of a stigma of being labelled as 'weak' being 'a girl' and not '[emotionally] strong enough' to be a paramedic, representing an underlying fear of threat in relation to their professional role, reputation and gender identity. Linguistically, such beliefs were articulated with a sense of 'we should just get on with it' because 'that's what we do' and a passive acceptance that trauma exposure is an unfortunate reality of the work. For Vix and Rebecca, these entrenched cultural beliefs became a significant barrier in preventing them from seeking support at a time when they most needed it. Interestingly, international studies such as that by Gouweloos-Trines et al.'s [29] study of 813 Australian prehospital providers identified similar cultural attitudes towards distress and emotional expression. However, the consideration of gendered discourse in terms of emotional display, dissonance and indeed, occupational mental health, has received little attention within paramedic research literature.

In contrast to the above, embodied within all of the participants' narratives was an acknowledgement that talking with and having the support of others was in fact extremely helpful, particularly in talking with close, trusted crewmates and colleagues. This promoted a sense of feeling connected to others, with a level of interpersonal shared understanding between those within the ambulance communities within which the participants worked. Despite concerns around emotional vulnerability, the narratives of several participants in this study alluded to a closed-knit culture which created psychosocial support and safety, that alleviated feelings of isolation, appeared to help with emotional regulation, feeling grounded and made the experience seem less overwhelming [30]. Talking provided new perspectives on the experience, from which developed new understandings and meanings about the incident and their personal reactions to it [23, 31]. Similar findings were also noted in other studies of emergency services workers [32–34].

Whilst a couple of the participants felt able to share their emotional experiences of distress with only a few close colleagues, the incident was for some, shared (within the confines of confidentiality) with a wider group of peers, with discussions held around the realities of clinical practice. Such conversations held a reflective space which facilitated exploration and discursive inquiry into any technical challenges encountered. This professional reflexion is by its very nature, generally unable to be provided by external supporters such as partners and family, who may be less familiar with the technical aspects of the work and the shared language and associated meanings used between ambulance personnel. Thus, to have an opportunity to defuse with colleagues in this way appears to be a unique experience which is unable to be provided with such connection by any other outlet. It offers subjective exploration which may help to normalise and authenticate one's position as a professional practitioner.

The traditional ritualistic practice of narrative-telling within emergency ambulance communities also offers opportunity to make practical sense of traumatic scenes and to offer a form of cultural normalisation of the incidents that individual ambulance personnel attend [35]. These practices may also act as a 'rite of passage' ([21], p. 735) whereby to have attended to such an incident and performed clinical skills is such that it develops an air of peer respect. Symbolically, this is socioculturally complex in defining one's professional identity, belonging, and collective acceptance within the peer group. However, this raises questions around informal hierarchies, power distribution and behaviours and beliefs which are deemed culturally acceptable [22]. Indeed, the practice of narrative-telling frames unspoken group rules and implicit assumptions around emotional display and expression. Although bound within the complexities of organisational culture, the use of symbolic language may, through outlets such as humour, be a way for ambulance personnel to indirectly express emotions safely within their closed cultural environment [36]. On the contrary, some individuals may experience anxieties and fears around their sense of integrity and ability to conform to these unwritten cultural norms when experiencing overwhelming emotions/distress. Importantly, Lazarsfeld-Jensen [21] wrote 'such attitudes lock paramedics into the world of other uniformed organisations that define their identity and culture on the basis of critical demands and shared trauma' [p. 738]. She added, 'these rites are like ancient rituals to exclude the weak from the work of the strong' [p. 738]. This certainly could be transposed into the rituals around emotional experiencing which were highlighted by Vix and Rebecca. This could lead to stigma and emotional dissonance, which in terms of trauma, may exacerbate any distress and lead to post-traumatic incident symptomology. Such a discourse around emotions and mental health may indeed, lead to the experiencing of internal incongruence between loyalty and external emotional conformity to group norms in comparison to one's internal felt emotional state. Subsequently, this can make it extremely challenging for individuals to seek psycho-emotional help and support.

Considering the psychosocial aspects of occupational culture within an ambulance service setting is of paramount importance in terms of post-traumatic distress, particularly given the influence that support and talking may have on mediating an individual's response to adverse events. Whilst the participants in this study shared their lived experiences and anxieties around communicating with others, it is critical to acknowledge that for some who experience post-traumatic distress, they may find it challenging to talk; they may not have the words to formulate a narrative of the event or have a reduced ability to recall details. Certainly, we know from neuropsychology that trauma exposure can affect cognitive function with disturbance to attention and concentration which influences an individual's ability to appraise and process information, or verbally express the memories that they hold.

Some individuals who encounter trauma may experience limited emotional awareness and not be able to recognise or describe their felt emotions or feel emotionally detached, which might be experienced as feeling numb [37]. This may negatively impact upon their ability to interpersonally relate or socially interact with others, particularly after trauma exposure where they are in a state of emotional hyperarousal and may be finding it more challenging to regulate their emotions. However, this is not to say that social affiliations are not important for these individuals – rather research indicates that experiencing trust, emotional warmth and support may have positive neurophysiological affects upon the 'basic aspects of the fear system' [38].

Whilst the psychosocial and emotional aspects of post-traumatic distress are hugely significant in terms of psychological wellbeing outcomes, a thorough examination in relation to the current study is beyond the scope of this chapter. Importantly however, a take-away point from this discussion is the importance of social experience and social bonds based on trust and shared norms in mediating how an individual responds to and experiences trauma, perceived threats and fears.

By providing psychosocial safety within reliable social networks such as ambulance communities, it may enable distressed individuals to regulate intense emotions including those of hyperarousal and resolve fears as they feel cared for, protected and reassured by the group. Intense emotions if left, may lead to re-experiencing, hypervigilance, avoidance and numbing, which are predictors for developing post-traumatic stress disorder. Thus, whilst the nature of ambulance work will not change, in that practitioners will be exposed to incidents which are psychologically distressing, informal social support can buffer an individual's psycho-emotional response and reduce the risk of developing post-traumatic sequelae.

The participants' positioning of the employing organisation as a psychological resource in times of vulnerability was an interesting aspect of this study's findings. Through language, it was viewed that affective commitment of the organisation to its employees in facilitating psychological wellbeing through perceived support was important to the participants and guided their self-beliefs upon their apparent value, worth and importance to the organisation; a finding also identified by Petrie et al. [39]. The commitment, willingness to listen and availability of managers appeared to provide those participants with emotional reassurance and reduce their feelings of distress. However, for the participants that did not receive the support that they needed, there were expressions of abandonment, feeling unvalued and a feeling of discontent and disconnection from managers. It is plausible that in their feelings of rejection, the participants were demonstrating an emotional attachment response to the organisation [40]. Indeed, from their study, Petrie et al. [39] found that the supportive behaviours of managers in creating psychosocial safety had a significant influence upon staff mental health.

Engaging with emotionality within ambulance organisations is a considered point within a few academic studies. From this phenomenological exploration of the participants' occupational life-world experiences, an underlying organisational discourse around mental wellbeing and post-incident psychosocial support was noted. This indicated an inherent, embedded view of individualisation, with a cultural belief that emotionality and distress were innately the concern of the beholder. This was conceptualised as 'within' an individual rather than understood in terms of external influences, such as socially constructed cultural ideologies whereby emotionality is created within the social discourse ascribed through group norms and beliefs. This was particularly apparent in terms of accepting help. It challenged individuals seeking assistance and accessing formal support such as counselling. For most of the participants, once they had overcome any internal conflict and courageously accessed therapy, they in the most part, found it beneficial and enhanced their wellbeing.

Social bonds extended beyond the familial sense of togetherness experienced within their occupational cultural groups, to include key others who were trusted and could provide emotional and practical support. It was apparent within their narratives that psycho-emotional overlap was present between participants' professional and private life-worlds. Some felt able to disclose their feelings and seek comfort from partners, non-ambulance friends and key others. Interestingly, several of the participants' partners were either paramedics or within the nursing/medical profession, so a level of shared understanding of distressing scenes was experienced. For others, however, disclosure led to frustration through feeling misunderstood or that those external to the ambulance service were unable to empathically comprehend what they had faced.

In addition, espoused within their accounts, was a need to provide psychosocial safety to their loved ones and friends, to protect them from the horrors and distress that they had witnessed, thus participants actively chose not to share some details/ feelings in an effort to save them from vicarious traumatisation. Participants talked of the impact of a loss of authenticity in relationships, which in the longer-term appeared to result in a loss of connection with friends and family members, narrowing their social support to those within the Service.

LIMITATIONS OF THE STUDY

It is recognised that the recruited cohort within this study was a specific occupational group and is limited in that those in other related positions (such as ambulance managers, non-clinicians or emergency call takers) were not included. The study was also limited to a single geographical area, primarily due to the research constraints associated with this academic work. Whilst the data collated were rich and detailed, the sample size was small, and the results are not generalisable.

CONCLUSION

Psychological trauma exposure is an inevitable reality of clinical practice within the context of emergency ambulance care. Through phenomenological inquiry, this study has intimately explored the psychosocial and emotional life-world experiences of six serving ambulance personnel, who had witnessed particularly distressing calls. The findings of the study highlight the ambiguity and complexity of inherent, intrinsic beliefs and norms associated with ambulance occupational culture and the impact this had upon the participants in terms of post-traumatic symptomology, cognitively processing the event and in accessing post-incident support.

Fundamentally, the thread linking all the themes was the need for psychosocial connectivity and psychological safety to promote a trusting environment in which the participants could share emotional authenticity and their narrative experience. Whilst individuality is key, and some prefer particular support mechanisms, the participants had shared commonalities in wishing to share with colleagues, particularly crew mates who had also experienced the same incident. Having the opportunity to defuse with managers was also highly valued and is consistent with previous research findings which note the influence of manager support in terms of mediating psychological distress responses. Critically, it was the opportunity to talk, to be listened to, heard and understood without judgement or criticism which was paramount. Through narrating the incident under these conditions, it appeared that the participants were using talking as a way of processing the traumatic memories that they held of the call, and this helped them to reconstruct meanings and make sense of their own reactions, their beliefs and views about what happened.

The findings highlight the complex dynamics within social and relational interactions experienced by the participants and suggest that a greater understanding and additional research are required into the nature and impact of psychological trauma exposure upon frontline ambulance workers. Recognition of the fundamental importance of talking and informal defusing between colleagues as well as more formal processes of support such as managerial advice and guidance, and psychotherapeutic interventions, cannot be underestimated in their role of mediating distress.

CONFLICTS OF INTEREST

There are no conflicts of interest associated with this author.

REFERENCES

1. Clompus, S. and Albarran, J.W. (2016). Exploring the nature of resilience in paramedic practice: a psychosocial study. *International Journal of Emergency Nursing* 28: 1–7.
2. Halpern, J., Maunder, R.G., Schwartz, B., and Gurevich, M. (2012). The critical incident inventory: characteristics of incidents which affect emergency medical technicians and paramedics. *BMC Emergency Medicine* 12: 10.
3. Knor, J., Pekara, J., Seblova, J. et al. (2020). Qualitative research of violent incidents toward young paramedics in the Czech Republic. *Western Journal of Emergency Medicine* 21 (2): 463–468.
4. Crown Prosecution Service (2020). Assaults on Emergency Workers (Offences) Act 2018. https://www.cps.gov.uk/legal-guidance/assaults-emergency-workers-offences-act-2018 (accessed 19 November 2020).
5. Heaney, C. (2020). Paramedics speak out against assault rate as staff told to delay treatment in the face of violence. https://www.abc.net.au/news/2020-01-18/paramedic-assaults-rising-northern-territory-st-johns-ambulance/11872420 (accessed 24 July 2020).
6. South Western Ambulance Service NHS Foundation Trust (2020). Ambulance service condems [hashtag]unacceptable assaults. https://www.swast.nhs.uk/welcome/latest-news/ambulance-service-condemns-unacceptable-assaults (accessed 24 July 2020).
7. Mishra, S., Goebert, D., Char, D. et al. (2010). Trauma exposure and symptoms of post-traumatic stress disorder in emergency medical services personnel in Hawaii. *Emergency Medicine Journal* 27: 708–711.
8. American Psychiatric Association (2013). *Diagnostic and Statistical Manual of Mental Disorders: Diagnostic and Statistical Manual of Mental Disorders*, 5e. Arlington, VA: American Psychiatric Association.
9. Pai, A., Suris, A.M., and North, C.S. (2017). Posttraumatic stress disorder in the DSM-5: controversy, change and conceptual considerations. *Behavioural Sciences* 7 (1): 7.
10. Davis, K., MacBeth, A., Warwick, R., and Chan, S.W.Y. (2019). Posttraumatic stress symptom severity, prevalence and impact in ambulance clinicians: the hidden extent of distress in the emergency services, traumatology. http://dx.doi.org/10.1037/trm0000191 (accessed 23 March 2020).

11. Fjeldheim, C.B., Nothling, J., Pretoruis, K. et al. (2014). Trauma exposure, posttraumatic stress disorder and the effect of explanatory variables in paramedic trainees. *BMC Emergency Medicine* 14: 11. https://doi.org/10.1186/1471-227X-14-11.

12. Halpern, J., Maunder, R.G., Schwartz, B., and Gurevich, M. (2014). Downtime after critical incidents in emergency medical technicians/paramedics. *Biomed Research International* https://www.hindawi.com/journals/bmri/2014/483140/ (accessed 24 March 2020).

13. Murray, E., Krahe, C., and Goodsman, D. (2018). Are medical students in prehospital care at risk of moral injury? *Emergency Medicine Journal* 35: 590–594.

14. Ward, C.L., Lombard, C.J., and Gwebushe, N. (2006). Critical incident exposure in south african emergency services personnel: prevalence and associated mental health issues. *Emergency Medicine Journal* 23 (3): 226–231.

15. Henckes, N. and Nurok, M. (2015). 'The First Pulse You Take is Your Own – But Don't Forget Your Colleagues' emotion teamwork in pre-hospital emergency medical services. *Sociology of Health and Illness* 37 (7): 1023–1038.

16. Lowery, K. and Stokes, M.A. (2005). Role of peer support and emotional expression on post-traumatic stress disorder in student paramedics. *Journal of Traumatic Stress* 18 (2): 171–179.

17. Joseph, S. (2011). *What Doesn't Kill Us: The New Psychology of Posttraumatic Growth*. London: Piatkus.

18. Hunt, N. and McHale, S. (2010). *Understanding Traumatic Stress*. Sheldon Press.

19. Deery, S.J., Iverson, R.D., and Walsh, J.T. (2010). Coping strategies in call centres: work intensity and the role of co-workers and supervisors. *British Journal of Industrial Relations* 48: 181–200.

20. McFarlane, A.C. and Bryant, R.A. (2007). PTSD in occupational settings: anticipating and managing the risk. *Occupational Medicine* 57: 404–410.

21. Lazarsfeld-Jensen, A. (2014). Telling stories out of school: experiencing the paramedic's oral traditions and role dissonance. *Nurse Education in Practice* 14: 734–739.

22. Tangherlini, T. (2000). Heroes and lies: storytelling tactics among paramedics. *Folklore* 111: 43–66.

23. Horowitz, M. (1986). *Stress Response Syndromes*, 2e. Northvale, NJ: Jason Aronson.

24. Scoglio, A.A.J., Rudat, D.A., Garvert, D. et al. (2018). Self-compassion and responses to trauma: the role of emotion regulation. *Journal of Interpersonal Violence* 33 (13): 2016–2036.

25. Miles, S. (2019). Addressing shame: what role does shame play in the formation of a modern medical professional identity? *Journal of Psychiatry Reform* 44 (1): 1–5.

26. Bennett, P., Williams, Y., Page, N. et al. (2005). Associations between organisational and incident factors: emotional distress in emergency ambulance personnel. *British Journal of Clinical Psychology* 44: 215–226.

27. Prati, G. and Pietrantoni, L. (2010). The relation of perceived and received social support to mental health among first responders: a meta-analytic review. *Journal of Community Psychology* 38 (3): 403–417.

28. Smith, A. and Roberts, K. (2003). Interventions for post-traumatic stress disorder and psychological distress in emergency ambulance personnel: a review of the literature. *Emergency Medicine Journal* 20: 75–78.

29. Gouweloos-Trines, J., Tyler, M.P., Giummarra, M.J. et al. (2017). Perceived support at work after critical incidents and its relation to psychological distress: a survey among prehospital providers. *Emergency Medicine Journal* 34: 816–822.

30. Lepore, S.J. (2001). A social-cognitive processing model of emotional adjustment to cancer. In: *Psychosocial Interventions for Cancer* (eds. A. Baum and B.L. Anderson), 96–116. Washington, DC: American Psychological Association.

31. Jonsson, A. and Segesten, K. (2003). The meaning of traumatic events as described by nurses in ambulance service. *Accident and Emergency Nursing* 11: 141–152.

32. Alexander, D.A. and Klein, S. (2001). Ambulance personnel and critical incidents. *British Journal of Psychiatry* 178: 76–81.

33. Essex, B. and Benz-Scott, L. (2008). Chronic stress and associated coping strategies among volunteer EMS personnel. *Prehospital Emergency Care* 12 (1): 69–75.

34. Regehr, C. and Millar, D. (2007). Situation critical: high demand, low control and low support in paramedic organisations. *Traumatology* 13: 49–58.

35. Granter, E., Wankhade, P., McCann, L. et al. (2019). Multi-dimensions of work intensity: ambulance work as edgework. *Work, Employment and Society* 33 (2): 280–297.

36. Regehr, C., Goldberg, G., and Hughes, J. (2002). Exposure to human tragedy, empathy and trauma in ambulance paramedics. *Americal Journal of Orthopsychiatry* 72 (4): 505–513.

37. Declercq, F., Vanheule, S., and Deheegher, J. (2010). Alexithymia and posttraumatic stress: subscales and symptom clusters. *Journal of Clinical Psychology* 66 (10): 1076–1089.

38. Charuvastra, A. and Cloitre, M. (2008). Social bonds and posttraumatic stress disorder. *Annual Review Psychology* 59: 301–328.

39. Petrie, K., Gayed, A., Bryan, B.T. et al. (2018). The importance of manager support for the mental health and wellbeing of ambulance personnel. *PLoS One* 13 (5): e0197802. https://doi.org/10.1371/journal.pone.0197802.

40. Halpern, J., Maunder, R.G., Schwartz, B., and Gurevich, M. (2011). Attachment insecurity, responses to critical incident distress and current emotional symptoms in ambulance workers. *Stress and Health* 28: 51–60.

PART 2

PRACTICE

CHAPTER 6

On Knowing, Not Knowing and Well-Being

Conversations About Practice

Clare Morris[1,2]

[1] Barts and The London School of Medicine and Dentistry, Queen Mary University of London, London, UK
[2] Institute of Continuing Education, University of Cambridge, Cambridge, UK

INTRODUCTION

This chapter explores the ways in which we approach conversations about practice, particularly the conversations we have when things do not go according to plan, when mistakes are made and when people find themselves in a place of not knowing what to do. This emphasis on *knowing* is a purposeful one, because the professions have long been defined by their claims to specialised knowledge, something that is argued to distinguish them from other occupational groups [1]. The continual development of a specialised knowledge base is at the very heart of medical and healthcare practice. The education of health professionals extends long beyond the heady graduation ceremonies that mark the end of an intense period of initial professional formation. New graduates enter the healthcare workforce with a dual worker-learner status that is maintained long after their transition into their chosen profession. As they join the clinics, wards and theatres, they work alongside other learner-workers such as the medical 'trainees' who may have already spent a decade or more further developing their specialist knowledge and practice. If a state of knowing is a defining characteristic of professional life and professional identity, what happens when we find ourselves in a state of not-knowing? The answer lies, at least in part, in how others around us respond.

The Mental Health and Wellbeing of Healthcare Practitioners: Research and Practice, First Edition.
Edited by Esther Murray and Jo Brown.

The healthcare workforce is defined by its professional boundaries, by hierarchical structures and power-relations. These relations are pivotal in career progression and success. They are pivotal too, in helping less experienced or expert practitioners make sense of the curriculum of the workplace, in order to develop their knowledgeable practice. Yet sadly we know that not all learning cultures are supportive cultures. Accounts of bullying, harassment, undermining, mistreatment and incivility are far too common in healthcare workplaces, something that sits so starkly against working practices where the raison d'être is the provision of compassionate care for others [2]. We know too that whilst conversations about practice are critical to ensuring safe, reflective practice, they are not always conducted in ways that achieve their desired aim.

This chapter provides an opportunity to think about the ways in which we support and develop healthcare professionals. The first section explores the inter-relationships between knowing, not-knowing and well-being. The second draws upon the last two decades of my own professional practice, working with healthcare professionals to help them develop their practice as educators and educational leaders. Here, I will explore approaches to supportive and developmental conversations, conversations that have the development of practice at their heart.

CONTEXT

Professional Learning and Well-Being

Whilst a detailed exploration of professional learning is beyond the scope of this chapter, articulating a standpoint on professional learning helps to make sense of the relationship between knowing, not knowing and well-being. I write from a socio-cultural viewpoint, a view on learning that goes beyond a singular focus on the acquisition of knowledge. Sociocultural theories see learning as part of everyday practice, as a social and relational act that involves processes of becoming (a professional) and belonging (to a profession) [3, 4]. Sociocultural theories invite consideration of the ways in which shared practice develops over time, influenced by history and culture i.e. 'the ways we do things around here'. It invites us to consider the ways in which *newcomers*, whether students, trainees or new, experienced co-workers, are invited to take part in a shared practice with others, developing not only their professional practice but their sense of professional identity [3]. Newcomers learn ways of thinking, talking and acting by taking part in those shared practices [5]. Learning is therefore seen as an embodied act as a newcomer is invited to make a meaningful contribution to shared work activity such as patient care.

Billett reminds us that this social and relational process is shaped by the interests, intentions and engagement of workers and learners. He reminds us too that

> *"Humans are subject to emotion, inconsistency in responses, exhaustion and inept responses."* [6]

It is perhaps unsurprising therefore that things can go wrong. Illing et al. for example, provide a stark account of bullying and harassment across the UK National Health Service, noting that the prevalence is higher in strongly hierarchical settings [2]. The consequences of bullying are far reaching, impacting on the psychological and physical health of both victims and onlookers. There are organisational consequences too – higher levels of sickness, lower levels of job satisfaction, higher levels of staff turnover and a negative impact on the quality of care provided [2]. Concerns about negative behaviours in healthcare workplaces are shared across the globe and are located across different professional groups and specialties [7–12].

Organisational Culture, Learning and Well-Being

Negative organisational cultures all too readily translate into negative learning cultures. For example, a study of the experiences of Australian nursing students showed that more than half had experienced some form of bullying or harassment in the past year of their clinical placements, from others within their own profession, including placement facilitators [7]. In the USA, it was noted that up to 20% of medical students across the country reported *mistreatment* each year, from within and beyond their professional group [8]. Mistreatment is defined as behaviour, whether intentional or unintentional, that shows 'disrespect for the dignity of others and unreasonably interferes with the learning process' [13]. The raising of a distinction between intended and unintended behaviours is an interesting one to consider. Harassment is also understood as unwanted or unwelcome behaviour that violates the dignity of another and that which creates a hostile environment [14]. The related loss of dignity may result in feelings of shame, an emotion that can have a significant and pervasive impact on self-esteem and therefore well-being.

Studies and accounts of shame in health professions education further illuminate relationships between knowing, not-knowing and well-being. Lindström explored medical students accounts of shame inducing situations during their clinical placements [9]. These included both first-hand and bystander accounts, for example witnessing situations where patients were treated in shame-inducing ways. Their first-hand accounts of shame were linked to 'being taken by surprise' or 'being exposed'. This included being required to undertake procedures they were not prepared for, in front of others and being verbally shamed for aspects of their practice in front of their peers and/or patients.

> "Students also related shame to the asymmetry of power in the positions of the people present and to the hierarchy of the medical culture, which produces inequalities" [9]

Whether intentional or otherwise, for these students, precious workplace learning opportunities focussed on their clinical practice and knowledge became shame inducing situations. Bynum explores the relationships between shame, guilt and medical learning, noting that shame can arise from making mistakes and from being wrong – forms of not knowing. Shame is a complex response that is linked to negative self-evaluations. For the person experiencing shame therefore, 'there is no distinction between the self and the behaviour' [15]. As educators, supervisors and mentors, we need to be extremely careful therefore that our conversations about practice remain focussed on practice not person. This includes those so-called throw-away comments about colleagues that involve profession or discipline stereotyping, that both undermine the work of our colleagues and stigmatise the care they provide [10, 16]. Bynum notes that guilt, unlike shame, does not have the same impact on self, perhaps because of its reparative potential. *In short, a person who experiences guilt may believe that* 'this thing I did was bad', *whereas someone experiencing shame believes* 'I am bad'. [15]

Learning to be a healthcare professional inevitably involves being in circumstances of not knowing, whether it is about knowing how or when to do something, or the reasons why one might do something. It is vital therefore that we find ways to teach, to foster and support development without shame. One might hope that 'teaching by humiliation' was a thing of the past, not one that some describe as a 'trans-generational' legacy in medical education and training [8, 11, 12]. Teaching by humiliation is often associated with bedside teaching methods based on questioning students and trainees to the point where they can no longer provide answers. This may go beyond the types of factual questions where there is a right answer, to those that the questioner believes to be the right answer, even where a range of possible approaches may co-exist [17]. Whilst there are merits in teaching through questioning, to develop clinical reasoning skills for example, it is important that it is done in ways that help the learner think and develop. As Mavis and colleagues note

> "When a reasonable person can tell that a student does not know the answers to questions, yet the faculty member continues to pepper the student with questions, the goal of the questions likely has shifted from assessment and teaching to humiliation and disgrace." [8]

Historically, this type of teaching has been defended on the grounds of being a rite of passage, one that somehow teaches valuable lessons. One might argue that it is only defensible if there is no other way to achieve the same, or indeed better outcomes, when clearly there are. Even when the questioner's intentions are positive, the consequences may be less so. This perhaps reflects what has been described as a negativity bias in health professions education; a negativity bias is a tendency to attend to negative experiences, a practice that may inadvertently be reinforced by popular teaching methods and feedback practices [18]. One example might be the use of high fidelity simulation, an innovative, powerful approach to health professional education, that has enabled the rehearsal of clinical practice in 'safe ways'; however, safety comes in many forms, not least in terms of the psychological safety of those who take part in simulations. Many of us have experienced the types of simulation scenarios that escalate rapidly to the point of catastrophic error, publicly broadcasting the participants' state of not-knowing to the onlookers. This can be further amplified by using debrief methods that inadvertently become an opportunity for uninvited group feedback to the participant, rather than one where the participant reflects on the learning for the shared benefit of those taking part. It is worth noting that an analysis of narratives from healthcare professional students taking part in simulation scenarios include descriptions of humiliation, linked to being unprepared, or under prepared for the scenario. For some, this was about the emotional aspects of their simulation experience being left unacknowledged in debrief [19]. There is no doubt that learning in simulation can have a powerful impact on performance and it provides opportunities for learning through making mistakes. Whilst much of healthcare education is focussed on the avoidance of errors, learning through deliberate error, that is by practising mistakes, can have a positive impact on learning, with positive transfer to patient care situations [20]. The challenge is to find ways where the psychological safety of participants is considered alongside the patient safety benefits of the teaching methods adopted.

Feelings of shame and inadequacy arise from many sources including from within; there is a growing literature on imposter syndrome in medicine, extending beyond periods of being in training. Imposter syndrome is characterised by feelings of inadequacy, where people doubt their practice and their ability, even in cases where they have had observable or tangible success. Imposter syndrome is linked with a fear of being 'found out' and is associated with pervasive self-doubt, anxiety and burnout [21]. A recent review of the literature on imposter syndrome in medicine showed associations with gender (being higher in women), in those with low self-esteem and those with strong desires for perfectionism [22]. The authors suggest that the culture of medical training may be a contributing factor, particularly in environments where help seeking can be construed as a sign of weakness, where not knowing something is a source of shame. The question arises therefore about how we can create a safe and supportive learning culture, one where

'people feel safe to speak up, dialogues take place about success, uncertainties, shame, fears and errors, and trainees and physicians work with compassion and empathy towards their patients, their colleagues and themselves' [21]

Implications for Educational Practice

How then do we create an environment where it is possible to talk about practice in ways that develop the practice and value the practitioner? In the remainder of this chapter I will focus on three different types of conversations. The first are conversations that allow us to learn from mistakes. The second type of conversations focus on learning through questioning. The final type of conversation is a developmental conversation, that is a conversation that has someone else's development in mind. This invites a reframing of debrief and feedback methods.

Learning from Mistakes

Mistakes are an inevitable part of professional life, openly discussing them may be less so. Training in error disclosure is too often part of the hidden curriculum of professional learning, with less experienced workers taking direction from the behaviours they see around them [23]. Negative role modelling of senior team members fosters unprofessional and unethical behaviours in others. This might be witnessing senior team members humiliate others for mistakes they have made or failing to accept responsibility for their own mistakes, seeking to shift the blame to others. Fortunately, we are more likely to experience positive role modelling and it is within every practitioners gift, accepting responsibility for an error, disclosing the error and apologising to patients and families where relevant [23]. This aligns to the earlier distinction between guilt and shame inducing situations; in following and modelling best practice around error disclosure, there is scope to lessen the impact on self-esteem and wellbeing. Discussing errors with colleagues can have a positive impact on professional relationships, particularly where it is possible to identify someone you believe will be a supportive listener if required. This is someone with whom you can discuss your emotional responses to the situation encountered, not just 'the facts' as may happen in more formal settings [24].

An ethnographic study of newly qualified nurses (*NQNs*) highlights learning from mistakes as one of four different types of 'invisible learning' in first posts, which also includes *learning from experience, informal learning from colleagues* and *muddling through* [25]. This invisible learning works best where the strategy operated by ward managers is one of 'safe challenge' i.e. one where the NQN is in a supportive environment and where the work they are delegated is that which can stretch them yet can be handled safely. A supportive environment here is one where the potential to make mistakes is acknowledged, where errors are pointed out (if need be) and discussed as learning opportunities. As the authors note

"Learning from challenging experiences can be extremely helpful to NQNs in building their confidence in being able to handle potentially frightening, challenging and emotionally stressful situations. However, without adequate support and reflective space, this opportunity for positive learning can have the opposite effect, increasing NQN fears and anxieties, and decreasing their confidence levels" [25]

Sadly, not all practitioners feel able to talk about mistakes and as many as one in ten do not feel they can identify a supportive listener from among their colleagues [26].

There is scope for what are typically informal conversations about practice, and mistakes in practice, to become formalised into everyday workplace structures, such as 'morbidity and mortality rounds' (*MMRs*). An ethnographic study of MMRs suggests that there is considerable scope to role model how experienced clinicians deal with difficult situations and outcomes, by 'worrying aloud' about errors, by accepting responsibility for mistakes made and by expressing sadness and frustration about events [27]. Trainees attending such rounds may not always recognise this as part of the curriculum of the workplace however, making the hidden curriculum more overt by signalling that this is a space where we work through mistakes together, where we support each other and spend time recognising the learning that can arise from our experiences is vital [28]. The increasing adoption of Schwartz rounds suggests that there is a move towards conversations about practice as an embodied practice, where emotional dimensions of learning are given as much space as the cognitive and behavioural [29].

Talking About Mistakes

- Make error disclosure practices an explicit part of the curriculum
- Be a positive role model – accept, disclose, apologise
- Adopt supervisory practices that offer challenge and support
- Talk openly about mistakes, including your own
- Attend to the affective dimensions of learning

Learning Through Questioning

A sociocultural stance on learning leads us to think about the ways in which we help newcomers to a profession or community begin to think, talk and act like members of that community [5]. How might we do this in ways that enable our learners to explore their knowing and not-knowing, to maintain their dignity, to develop their thinking and practice? A move from teaching by humiliation to learning by example?

We might look into strategies that foster the development of clinical reasoning skills, classically approached by teaching through questioning. Rather than posing questions designed to elicit facts (assessment type questions), we might pose questions that allow a collective exploration of *possible* explanations, *possible* options for action. Studies have shown that the use of self-explanation (or think-aloud) techniques using hypothetical or 'paper-cases' can have a positive impact on the clinical reasoning skills deployed when meeting real patients [30, 31]. Clinicians think-aloud methods model how experienced practitioners weigh up information in order to formulate plans for action. Rather than saying 'the best way is this' or 'my preference is that', the clinician-educator might say

> "I am weighing up X over Y. My experience leads me to think X is perhaps the best way forward, but my instinct is leading me to consider Y because of this particular factor in their history or examination".

Likewise, they might encourage learners to 'think aloud' when it comes to formulating a diagnosis or treatment plan. Similar methods can be used with 'real' cases, modelling the ways in which clinicians make and justify decisions on a daily basis.

This explicit emphasis on the thinking behind actions taken allows an analytical stance when outcomes are not as anticipated. Effective clinician-educators use prompts as well as questions when fostering this kind of thinking. They might ask questions like 'what principle is being applied here' or 'how does this relate to what you already know' or 'where have you seen something similar before' or 'in what ways is this similar or different to what you already know about X'. The use of prompts to encourage reflection amplifies the value of self-explanation alone [30].

> **Tips for Learning Through Questioning**
> - Adopt clinician 'think aloud' methods to model your own reasoning
> - Encourage exploration of a range of possible approaches before anchoring on a preferred approach
> - Move beyond 'what' type (assessment) questions to those that foster deeper thinking and analysis, such as what if, when might, how might etc.
> - Use prompts to foster reasoning skills

Learning Through Debrief and Feedback

In earlier sections of this chapter, we explored the unintended consequences of teaching methods that took learners by surprise, that left them feeling exposed, that failed to acknowledge emotional dimensions of learning situations. We looked too at how these situations can lead to feelings of shame that fail to distinguish between practice and person, where doing a bad thing becomes being a bad person [15]. In this final section, the focus is on the ways in which we might approach conversations about practice, whether with our learners, with those we supervise, those we work alongside. The emphasis is upon feedback practices, re-framed here as developmental conversations, that is a conversation that has another person's development in mind.

To start with, it is helpful, in my mind at least, to distinguish between debriefing and feedback in health professions education. Debriefing is often used following learning experiences in simulation but is a commonly adopted strategy in postgraduate training, at the end of a clinic, or theatre list, for example. Debriefing is a term with military origins, to debrief someone is to question them, typically following a completed mission or undertaking. The person returning from the mission provides a vivid account of what they experienced, drawing on all the senses so that others might gain 'inside information' to inform their shared next steps. What might that mean if adopted as a teaching method in health professions education? It would mean, perhaps, that the lived experience of one team member is offered up to the whole group as a shared resource for learning. By inviting the learner to provide a narrative account, which includes affective responses to their experiences (whether of simulated or actual experiences) they are offering a gift to the group. Together they analyse ways of responding. Together they seek to make connections between the shared experience and their own. Together they identify the learning arising from the scenario that they each can benefit from. This kind of debrief would be particularly powerful when bringing teams in to analyse existing practices and try out new ways of working to enhance patient care. This is rather different than what sometimes becomes a group feedback session, with observers free to comment on their peers' performance and how it may or may not be 'improved'.

So, what are the implications of re-framing feedback as a developmental conversation? Well the first is to emphasise dialogue, the fact that this is a *conversation* between two practitioners. It is however, a very particular conversation, shaped to greater or lesser extents by shared history, organisational culture and power relations [32]. This latter point is important, no matter how well intentioned and supportive your feedback may be, how it is received, and therefore acted upon, will be shaped by a myriad of factors. One of these is to do with your credibility, in the eyes of the recipient. Where your practice is respected, where your approach to care is valued, the person receiving feedback is much more likely to act upon it [33]. So, one of the factors to consider when offering to give feedback to a colleague, is whether you are the person best placed to give that feedback. Choice and consent are seldom discussed in the context of feedback. Asking your colleague or learner if they would welcome a conversation about their practice is a starting point, even better if they set the agenda and ground rules of how, where and when that conversation happens. Ajjawi and Regehr offer a helpful definition of feedback in education, arguing 'the term feedback should be reserved for a dynamic and co-constructive process in a shared social or cultural space' [34]. They go on to explain that it is a collaborative approach, involving joint problem framing and the generation of shared understandings and solutions.

The second point of emphasis is upon the word *development*, that is a conversation that has someone else's development in mind. Too often 'feedback' conversations become an assessment conversation, where one person offers an analysis of what has gone before, yet spends little time talking about what might happen next. If the conversation is to be helpful, there has to be scope to explore different possibilities for action, authentically. In other words, to invite some shared thinking about ways to develop practice, recognising that the person best placed to decide on the way forward is the practitioner themselves. One of the ways to increase the usefulness of feedback is to see it as an ongoing dialogue, rather than a one-off encounter [32]. If a conversation has generated ideas about ways to develop practice, follow this through. This might be a simple check in, to see how things are going, or something more formalised, where you arrange to do some shared or observed practice.

How then to approach this developmental conversation? What strategies might we adopt? The answer does not lie in the use of particular models, however well intentioned, as there is no evidence to suggest that this makes a difference to how feedback is received and acted upon [32]. One of the risks of commonly adopted models, such as Pendleton's Rules, is they can be reductionist and arbitrarily divide practice into good and bad, strengths and weaknesses. There are two pitfalls here. Firstly, we know that feelings of shame leave little room for distinctions between practice and person. Binary distinctions of desirable or less desirable practice carry value judgements that too easily translate into the personal. It is important to avoid the use of judgemental language that may induce feelings of humiliation or shame [15, 35]. Secondly, these divisions of complex practice into graded categories belie the complexity of clinical work, the nuanced aspects of practice, including the fact there may be a range of possible responses to any one situation.

What might a developmental conversation look like? Well, many of the models classically adopted rely on the fact they are based upon 'constructive criticism'. Criticism again implies some degree of value judgement, a corrective type of response. Thinking about feedback as being a practice based upon critique rather than criticism may be more helpful here. Critique involves bringing together varied sources of information or evidence and coming up with an analysis. This feels like a more appropriate place to start a conversation about observed performance. The emphasis on observed performance is intentional as it is much more powerful to have a conversation about something where there has been a shared experience or a shared gaze than one that relies on second-hand information reported by a third party. Of course, if the conversation is about a specific incident, the practitioners themselves are well placed to offer a narrative account of what they experienced as the basis for further conversation. The emphasis on observed behaviours and actions maintains emphasis on practice not practitioner.

If you are invited to offer a commentary on performance (to 'give' feedback), there are some strategies that you may wish to consider adopting. The first is to utilise a simple 'what went well' and 'even better if' approach. This places emphasis on successful aspects of performance (too often overlooked because of the aforementioned negativity bias) yet offers suggestions about things that could be added to the repertoire of performance. You can make this more conversational by prefacing this with 'Well, for me, the way you did X, Y and Z was particularly effective/impressive because. . .' and invite a response in terms of the practitioners own critique, such as 'what about you, what were you particularly pleased about. . .' before moving onto suggestions for how they might enhance performance following the 'even better if' principle. This might be something like 'If I had any suggestions for things that might enhance your approach, I might focus on the way you did.. . .'

The other simple strategy to adopt is the 'When, then, I' approach. Here you start by describing the behaviour your observed and your analysis of its impact e.g. 'when you did X, (then) I could see the patient visibly relaxing' or 'when you said Y,(then) I noticed the patient became increasingly agitated'. The third element is where you share your own response to the situation, ideally in ways that prompt a reflective response in your colleague. 'When you did X, (then), I noticed that the patient became increasingly agitated, I wonder if there might have been a different way to explain what was happening?' Phrases like *I wonder, I am curious, I was concerned, I find it helpful to.* . . may invite further discussion about approaches adopted and how they might be adapted. The use of 'I' (rather than you) is important here, as it makes it clear that you recognise there may be other ways to view or approach the situation. The use of you too easily leads into conversations that imply criticism or judgement, even if that is not the intention.

Feedback as a Developmental Conversation

- Focus on practice not person
- Recognise feedback as a conversation that is influenced by context, culture and power differentials: seek consent to have the conversation.
- Reframe feedback as a conversation that has someone else's development in mind: ask what would be useful or helpful, do not assume.
- Generate options for possible next steps together: feedback as an ongoing dialogue involving follow up and follow through
- Move away from binary divisions of performance to an authentic narrative that focuses on development of practice

CONCLUDING COMMENTS

Healthcare practice is a complex practice. It is inevitable that practitioners will find themselves in positions of knowing and of not knowing. How they and we respond is pivotal when it comes to issues of self-belief, self-esteem and well-being. Conversations about practice in all its forms need to become part of the curriculum of the workplace. As practitioners, there is scope to role model the kind of behaviours that allow for the development of professional practice within an open and supportive culture. This includes modelling not-knowing, being open about mistakes and talking about the emotional aspects of practice. As a mentor, supervisor or educator, it means creating spaces for authentic conversations that offer both support and challenge: conversations that enable others to visit, revisit and rehearse alternative options for practice.

REFERENCES

1. Young, M. and Knowledge, M.J. (2014). *Expertise and the Professions*. Oxon: Routledge.
2. Illing, J., Carter, M., Thompson, N.J. et al. (2013). *Evidence Synthesis on the Occurrence, Causes, Consequences, Prevention and Management of Bullying and Harrassing Behaviours to Inform Decision Making in the NHS*. NHS National Institute for Health Research.
3. Lave, J. and Wenger, E. (1991). *Situated learning: Legitimate Peripheral Participation*. Cambridge: Cambridge University Press.
4. Wenger, E. (1998). *Communities of Practice*. Cambridge: Cambridge University Press.
5. Morris, C. (2012). Re-imagining 'the firm': clinical placements as time spent in communities of practice. In: *Work Based Learning in Clinical Settings—Insights from Socio-Cultural Perspectives* (eds. V. Cook, C. Daly and M. Newman). Oxford: Radcliffe Medical.
6. Billett, S. (2007). Including the missing subject. Placing the personal within the community. In: *Communities of Practice Critical Perspectives* (eds. J. Hughes, N. Jewson and L. Unwin), 55–57. London: Routledge.

7. Budden, L.M., Birks, M., Cant, R. et al. (2017). Australian nursing students' experience of bullying and/or harassment during clinical placement. *Collegian* 24 (2): 125–133.

8. Mavis, B., Sousa, A., Lipscomb, W., and Rappley, M.D. (2014). Learning about medical student mistreatment from responses to the medical school graduation questionnaire. *Academic Medicine* 89 (5): 705–711.

9. Lindström, U.H., Hamberg, K., and Johansson, E.E. (2011). Medical students' experiences of shame in professional enculturation. *Medical Education* 45 (10): 1016–1024.

10. Hoskison, K. and Beasley, B.W. (2019). A conversation about the role of humiliation in teaching: the ugly, the bad, and the good. *Academic Medicine* 94 (8): 1078–1080.

11. Barrett, J. and Scott, K.M. (2018). Acknowledging medical students' reports of intimidation and humiliation by their teachers in hospitals. *Journal of Paediatrics and Child Health* 54 (1): 69–73.

12. Scott, K.M., Caldwell, P.H., Barnes, E.H., and Barrett, J. (2015). "Teaching by humiliation" and mistreatment of medical students in clinical rotations: a pilot study. *Medical Journal of Australia* 203 (4): 185.

13. Colleges AoAM (2011). Medical school graduation questionnaire (GQ). https://www.aamc.org/data/gq/ (accessed 2 February 2021).

14. ACAS (2014). Bullying and harassment at work. A guide for managers and employers. (accessed 2 February 2021).

15. Bynum, W.E. IV and Goodie, J.L. (2014). Shame, guilt, and the medical learner: ignored connections and why we should care. *Medical Education* 48 (11): 1045–1054.

16. Ajaz, A., David, R., Brown, D. et al. (2016). BASH: badmouthing, attitudes and stigmatisation in healthcare as experienced by medical students. *BJPsych Bulletin* 40 (2): 97–102.

17. Kost, A. and Chen, F.M. (2015). Socrates was not a pimp: changing the paradigm of questioning in medical education. *Academic Medicine* 90 (1): 20–24.

18. Haizlip, J., May, N., Schorling, J. et al. (2012). Perspective: the negativity bias, medical education, and the culture of academic medicine: why culture change is hard. *Academic Medicine* 87 (9): 1205–1209.

19. Bearman, M., Greenhill, J., and Nestel, D. (2019). The power of simulation: a large-scale narrative analysis of learners' experiences. *Medical Education* 53 (4): 369–379.

20. Dyre, L., Tabor, A., Ringsted, C., and Tolsgaard, M.G. (2017). Imperfect practice makes perfect: error management training improves transfer of learning. *Medical Education* 51 (2): 196–206.

21. Atherley, A. and Meeuwissen, S.N.E. (2020). Time for change: overcoming perpetual feelings of inadequacy and silenced struggles in medicine. *Medical Education* 54 (2): 92–94.

22. Gottlieb, M., Chung, A., Battaglioli, N. et al. (2020). Impostor syndrome among physicians and physicians in training: a scoping review. *Medical Education* 54 (2): 116–124.

23. Martinez, W., Hickson, G.B., Miller, B.M. et al. (2014). Role-modeling and medical error disclosure: a national survey of trainees. *Academic Medicine* 89 (3): 482–489.

24. Luu, S., Patel, P., St-Martin, L. et al. (2012). Waking up the next morning: surgeons' emotional reactions to adverse events. *Medical Education* 46 (12): 1179–1188.

25. Allan, H.T., Magnusson, C., Evans, K. et al. (2016). Delegation and supervision of healthcare assistants' work in the daily management of uncertainty and the unexpected in clinical practice: invisible learning among newly qualified nurses. *Nursing Inquiry* 23 (4): 377–385.

26. Kaldjian, L.C., Forman-Hoffman, V.L., Jones, E.W. et al. (2008). Do faculty and resident physicians discuss their medical errors? *Journal of Medical Ethics* 34 (10): 717–722.

27. Kuper, A., Nedden, N.Z., Etchells, E. et al. (2010). Teaching and learning in morbidity and mortality rounds: an ethnographic study. *Medical Education* 44 (6): 559–569.

28. Benassi, P., MacGillivray, L., Silver, I., and Sockalingam, S. (2017). The role of morbidity and mortality rounds in medical education: a scoping review. *Medical Education* 51 (5): 469–479.

29. The Point of Care Foundation. About schwartz rounds. https://www.pointofcare foundation.org.uk/our-work/schwartz-rounds/about-schwartz-rounds/ Undated (accessed 2 February 2021).

30. Chamberland, M., Mamede, S., St-Onge, C. et al. (2015). Self-explanation in learning clinical reasoning: the added value of examples and prompts. *Medical Education* 49 (2): 193–202.

31. Chamberland, M., St-Onge, C., Setrakian, J. et al. (2011). The influence of medical students' self-explanations on diagnostic performance. *Medical Education* 45 (7): 688–695.

32. Lefroy, J., Watling, C., Teunissen, P.W., and Brand, P. (2015). Guidelines: the do's, don'ts and don't knows of feedback for clinical education. *Perspectives on Medical Education* 4 (6): 284–299.

33. Watling, C., Driessen, E., van der Vleuten, C.P.M., and Lingard, L. (2012). Learning from clinical work: the roles of learning cues and credibility judgements. *Medical Education* 46 (2): 192–200.

34. Ajjawi, R. and Regehr, G. (2019). When I say. . . feedback. *Medical Education* 53 (7): 652–654.

35. Bynum, W.E. IV (2015). Filling the feedback gap: the unrecognised roles of shame and guilt in the feedback cycle. *Medical Education* 49 (7): 644–647.

CHAPTER 7

The Complex Issues that Lead to Nurses Leaving the Emergency Department

Imogen Skene

Queen Mary University of London, London, UK

CONTEXT

Increasing Pressure

The National Health Service (*NHS*) is the biggest employer in Europe, employing 1.3 million people across the health service in England [1]. The performance of any healthcare system ultimately depends on the people working within it. The NHS is under increasing pressure, with 24.8 million attendances in the Emergency Department (*ED*) in 2018–2019, this is an increase of 21% since 2009–2010 [2]. Nurses are bound to feel the effects of this. Without a comparative increase in staffing and resources, there will be problems in dealing with this ever-increasing demand on the health service, which will inevitably impact on those working within it.

Nursing Shortages

Nursing shortages have been identified as a major factor in workforce issues in health-care systems. The vacancy rate in England for nursing is 11% with 41 722 posts vacant [3]. The impact of this is felt acutely by nurses, who have to manage an increasing workload with a reduced workforce, or with the support of agency nurses who may not be familiar with the department. This can contribute to nurses feeling burnt out, as well as a decrease in job satisfaction and a loss of opportunities for

The Mental Health and Wellbeing of Healthcare Practitioners: Research and Practice, First Edition.
Edited by Esther Murray and Jo Brown.

training and development. Working conditions are the top cited reason for nurses leaving the profession [4]. It is vital to establish the needs of nurses and provide support and development for their well-being and ultimately to retain them.

There are always a background number of vacancies as staff move between employers and advance their careers, but the current number requires addressing urgently [3]. This is recognised in the NHS long-term plan [1], with the aim to ensure a sufficient supply of nurses to address the shortages, but this involves both training new nurses and retaining those already in employment.

Workforce Retention

Workforce challenges have now overtaken funding as the greatest threat facing the NHS in England [5]. There is now a governmental focus on improving retention so that staff actively wants to stay working in the NHS. The 2019 Conservative manifesto [6] pledges 50 000 more nurses; this includes the retention of 18 500 nurses already employed in the NHS who would normally leave. This pledge therefore highlights a commitment for improving working conditions to achieve this increase in retention and help to retain experienced nurses in the NHS. Part of this retention plan may be achieved by the increase in funding for professional development which may boost staff morale.

The challenges of high vacancy rates, particularly in acute environments, such as the ED, lead to increased stresses and pressures on those in permanent positions. High vacancy rates lead to shifts being filled by bank or agency workers who may not be familiar with the environment and require time to orientate, they may also not be able to work in all areas of an ED, for example resus or triage which require additional skills and familiarity with the department. This is characterised by the term 'vicious circle'; as the scenario where high vacancy rates lead to an over reliance on agency nurses, which lead to an increased responsibility and burden for permanent staff, who are then attracted to less burdensome posts, but in doing so contribute to the increased burden on the remaining staff [7]. This highlights the importance of breaking the 'vicious circle' and improved retention of skilled and experienced staff.

Well-being

Staff well-being is the fourth highest priority for emergency medicine of the James Lind Alliance Priority Setting Partnership, which was constituted following extensive consultation with patients, public and carers [8]. This recognises that patients place a high priority upon ensuring nurses caring for them are happy and satisfied with their jobs. There is an increasing awareness of the negative psychological impact of providing emergency care. The Royal College of Nursing (RCN) has highlighted that the need for emotional support at any stage in the emergency nurse's career should never be underestimated. To support emergency nurses develop resilience, the RCN Competency framework aims to support nurses in exploring their experiences, to enable reflection and learning [9]. This framework provides a structure which supports nurses aiming to stay in emergency nursing.

Nurses who work in demanding areas such as the ED are likely to spend a considerable time working and being involved in intense interaction with people all day [10]. The nature of emergency care is physically demanding, and nursing staff are faced with meeting significant demands from high turnover and high acuity patients [11]. A potential consequence of such caring work is a negative and profound effect on emergency nurse's health that can be referred to as secondary traumatic stress [12]. Secondary traumatic stress may occur after daily exposure to witnessing trauma in conjunction with eliciting an empathic response. The nature of the workload is only intensifying; therefore, nurses need to be equipped to manage the challenges of this role.

Health and well-being in the workplace has been identified as an area for improvement in the NHS long-term plan [1], acknowledging that the best solutions come from the staff themselves. A number of the key messages and suggestions for improvements come from staff as they leave the department.

DESCRIPTION

Over the last decade I have worked in a number of EDs across the globe, as both an ED nurse and an ED clinical research nurse. This experience has given me a wealth of knowledge on the reasons why nurses leave the ED. In the following pages I will outline what I have discovered from conducting exit interviews with ED nurses.

There are many reasons why nurses move on from an ED. These include a desire for change, professional development, personal development, personal circumstances, for example a desire to travel, family life or moving to find affordable housing. However, there are also some negative contributing factors e.g. the impact of the shift work required in the ED, the burnout from the challenging pace of the department, the emotional impact of the challenging caseload, the departmental/organisational culture may also speed up the departure of those who might otherwise stay.

Exit Interviews

Exit interviews are a popular method for discovering reasons why people leave. Information from these interviews can also assist in identifying themes and problem areas. However, it is acknowledged in the literature [13] that exit interviews can be skewed as employees do not want to leave on a bad note, and consequently their reasons for resignation may not be entirely truthful. Therefore how, when and with whom the exit interview is conducted may influence the responses given. My aims in conducting exit interviews in the ED were primarily to identify themes which could be acted upon to improve retention. While there is no evidence to support the value of exit interviews in the reduction of turnover [13], I feel it is intuitively right to be aware of why staff members are leaving in order to be able to act and make improvements.

Why Do Nurses Leave the ED?

There are many reasons why nurses leave the ED – a promotion, a change of direction, a change of location to name but a few. There are normally a number of factors that have contributed to this decision including fatigue from shift work, a need for a change of place, the desire to provide a different type of care and a desire for further development. However, it often feels like a difficult decision has been taken, as when nurses leave, they often comment on their love of the camaraderie and teamwork that occurs in the department.

Nurses in the ED are exposed to emergency situations or critical states of illness and injury, particularly those working in major trauma centres. Because of the nature of this work, these occurrences are regular and ongoing. This ongoing exposure can lead to post traumatic stress, burnout fatigue and coping difficulties. There is currently little research focus on the effects of trauma on ED nurses or the needs of nurses to increase coping. In a study investigating secondary traumatic stress in EDs, it was found that 75% of nurses reported at least one secondary traumatic stress symptom in the last week [14]. Resuscitation and death were identified as influencing factors, and this correlated with the events reported in the exit interviews. These traumatic events can contribute to nurses leaving the ED, or needing a break [15].

Stress

Work-related stress is considered one of the biggest occupational health problems in the UK [16], with reports of high levels of work-related stress amongst healthcare professions [17]. UK-based occupation analysis has also demonstrated that nurses are among those in the work force who fall into a high stress category [18–20]. The RCN Employment survey in 2019 found that 63% of nurses felt they were under too much pressure at work and 61% were too busy to provide the level of care they would like [21].

Strategies are required to balance the stress of the time pressures that nurses face in the ED. There is a continuous need to balance the ability to provide care to patients and respond to the next. Nurses can feel divided in the provision and responding to care needs in a busy department; this is due to perceived time pressures which impact the communication style and perceived caring relationship [22]. It has been reported that approximately one third of nurses in an ED setting met the criteria for post-traumatic stress disorder [12]. Departments need effective leadership to foster a culture of staff well-being. This helps to balance the stress of time pressures.

Burnout

The term 'burnout' is used to describe workers reactions to chronic stress in occupations involving numerous direct interactions with people [23]. Burnout is especially common in caring professions such as healthcare, social work and teaching, with a prevalence of up to 25% in these professions [24]. Burnout amongst nurses seems to be on the rise and this is causing problems not only for the individuals involved, but also the NHS which is already stretched and now at risk of losing more staff. In a recent survey of ED staff 42.2% of respondents reported that they felt burnt out at work, 76% felt at 'high-risk' of future burnout within the following six months [25]. ED nurses are at high risk of burnout due to the increasing workload, shift patterns and inability to maintain personal well-being.

There are a number of factors which can contribute to occupational burnout; in general, people are at high risk of occupational burnout when they do not feel fully in control of their work. The ability to manage a workload is key. In the ED, the rota, patient flow and service demand can impact this. The combination of routine work interspersed with complex emotionally demanding tasks place ED nurses at a higher risk of burnout. Burnout is typically characterised by emotional exhaustion, deper-sonalisation and reduced personal accomplishment [11]:

a. Emotional exhaustion – is a feeling of being emotionally overextended by one's work. Exhaustion has an impact on the ability to carry out work safely, and also carries over into the personal life of the burnout sufferer, affecting rela-tionships and ability to have a fulfilling life outside of work.
b. Depersonalisation – is described as an unfeeling, unempathic and impersonal response to the interaction with patients.
c. Reduced personal accomplishment – relates to a sense of competence or achievement in ones work which results in job satisfaction, or if absent, dissatisfaction.

The toll of working in a busy ED can lead to nurses looking for a break, either from the ED or nursing altogether. This is particularly apparent when combined with the stress of working additional hours, while consolidating new knowledge and ensuring development milestones are reached (i.e. RCN competency framework).

While nurses leaving the ED are not all going to be burnt out, they often describe some of the elements of burnout – particularly the absent sense of accomplishment. Nurses describe feeling like they are providing care below the standard they would like to provide. This is echoed by the RCNs recent employment survey which shows six out of ten nurses say they cannot provide the level of care they want to [21]. Nurses are often motivated by the love of the job, the teamwork and the satisfaction of giving good care to patients and there is an emotional toil of not being able to provide that level of care.

Moral Injury

Nurses often spoke of a clinical case or where external factors limited their ability to provide care to their desired standard which affected their emotional well-being. This had an impact for months after the event. The term 'moral injury' is appropriate in some of these instances and is useful in conceptualising the psychological effects resulting from witnessing events which transgress their deeply held beliefs [26].

The term 'moral injury' has emerged from work with military veterans and can occur in response to acting or witnessing behaviours that go against an individual's values and moral beliefs [27]. A number of nurses leaving, mentioned being troubled by scenes that they had witnessed, both in terms of the nature of the event and in hospitals management. There was a sense of frustration about long bed waits for palliative and elderly patients and caring for patients in corridors. Rumination on the event has previously been identified as a major theme following trauma at work – nurses remembered the event and questioned their role and performance [15]. Situations that have been identified as a stress trigger in the literature include paediatric and geriatric abuse and injuries from avoidable situations and 'senseless' deaths [28]. This resonated with findings following interviews with pre-hospital medical students who in particular found cases with violent connotations hardest to process [26].

There are increasing concerns about overcrowding, with 'corridor care' becoming normal in EDs. With the growing demand on emergency services, and the expectation that departments will cope with the ever-increasing number of patients that arrive in the department at any one time, it is likely that this will contribute to moral injury in the providers. An article in the Guardian quotes Dr Adrian Boyle, the vice-president of the Royal College of Emergency Medicine, which represents A&E doctors, saying: 'Looking after people in corridors is demoralising and shameful for staff. People do feel that it's a failure when they have to look after people in corridors' [29].

The emotional repercussions of dealing with acutely unwell patients can be substantial. Emotional aspects of care are referred to as emotional labour, for nursing this can involve smiling and talking to patients in a calming voice even though they are anxious or worried [30]. It is used to make patients feel safe and is part of the normal routine of nursing [31]. Unfortunately, the nature of the ED, gives little time to debrief or reflect on events before needing to move on to the next job. Compassion fatigue and burnout can result.

Debrief

The ability to debrief is considered an important part of dealing with the events occurring in the ED. It is a way to discuss unanticipated outcomes, identify opportunities for improvement and to heal as a group. There are a number of ways to debrief, including 'hot' and 'cold' debriefs. A 'cold debrief' is where individuals or teams are provided with feedback sometime after the event, and is usually associated with improvements in process and patient outcome, whereas a 'hot debrief' is where the individuals or teams are debriefed immediately after the event [32]. Debrief has been shown to decrease professional stress and improve concentration, morale and work engagement [33]. However further work is required to ensure that debriefs are both able to happen at an appropriate time in the ED setting and in how they are conducted.

Most participants, in a study conducted in three EDs in Ireland, reported debriefing to occur after major incidents, such as major trauma, paediatric or traumatic deaths [33]. However, in major trauma centres, where these events occur on a regular basis, what is the best way to ensure there is opportunity to debrief and maintain staff well-being?

It is important to ensure there are the right psychological resources available to support staff in constructive debriefs, not only after traumatic events, but also for those who are experiencing high stress levels. Ensuring the culture of the department encourages this support, will help staff feel they can access these services. For some departments, having access to a clinical psychologist for staff who are regularly exposed to traumatic events, on top of everyday stressors including overcrowding and corridor nursing, has potential to improve well-being in a department.

Culture

The culture of a department is highly important. Valuing staff helps to build a culture that fosters satisfaction and retention [34]. The sense of teamwork and camaraderie is significant to the ED. People are social creatures and we need a team around us to support and champion us through the ups and downs of an ED. Having a social support network has been shown to be associated with resilience and is considered a protection from work-related stress [26]. If the culture is not supportive, working in the ED can also be isolating with antisocial shift patterns. The sense of cohesiveness was identified as a positive factor in a US study from a level 1 trauma centre [28]. The importance of co-worker support was identified in a study conducted on doctors in Canada and was associated with well-being [35]. At a senior level, social support at work from senior nurses and management plays an important role in the nurses' ability to cope [36]. Having good relationships with your co-workers, seniors and multidisciplinary team will improve the department culture and the satisfaction of those working in it.

Having support and role models who actively show an appreciation of staff is critical in sustaining a caring culture. Positive aspects of ED nursing include the knowledge of contributing to saving lives and making a difference [28]. Feeling a lack of appreciation by patients, their families or the organisation can contribute to workplace stress.

Shift Work

Rota and shift patterns are often cited as reasons for leaving the department. An ED nurse typically works 50% of shifts as anti-social hours (evenings, night shifts and weekends) due to the nature of the service. In England 12.5 hours shifts are common, whereas in Australia and New Zealand, eight hours shifts are more typical. Past studies of nurses and physicians have shown night shift work is a major factor in career dissatisfaction, burnout, work-family conflict and dysphoria [18, 37]. The impact of shift work is well documented. For example, a study found that shifts over 13 hours were linked to patient dissatisfaction in part due to poorer communication from the nurses and not receiving help as quickly as they wanted [37]. ED nurses typically work consecutive long shifts and as a result often feel fatigued which may contribute to a reduced productivity and impaired personal well-being.

The ability to have a good quality of life is also a factor. This includes having time for oneself, interests outside of work, family and a healthy and active lifestyle [35]. Whilst this is still possible while working in an ED, the sense of control (or the lack of it) may impact this – for example how far in advance the rota is provided, ability to plan and request time off.

Career Progression and Development

One of the reasons people leave is that they are looking for career development and progression. In the ED, this may be into roles such as practice education, clinical research, management or clinical progression, or roles such as advanced clinical practitioners. If this is not available in their current department, they will look further afield for new opportunities.

Nurses often mention a sense of accomplishment and achievement from the developmental opportunities that have occurred during an ED job – for example advanced assessment skills and skills in caring for patients with severe injuries. However, these need to be supported by formal training and further training is required as nurses progress in their ED roles.

Health Education England (HEE) has committed to increase the proportion of the budget for workforce development [1] and support from employers is key to ensure staff members are given the time to develop their skills. If staff members do not have support to develop these skills, this can contribute to dissatisfaction and burnout.

There is an old English proverb saying 'a change is as good as a rest', which means developing your professional interests can be as beneficial as taking a break. Enabling staff to take secondments and development opportunities may help staff members renew their interest in their line of work. Offering developmental opportunities, such as advanced training or secondments, has the potential to deliver a high return on the investment. It offers the career progression to motivate them to stay within the department and, just as importantly, equips them with skills to operate at an advanced level of professional practice and meet the needs of the patients.

For those progressing within emergency nursing, the RCN Competency framework was developed to provide a clear career structure. Key to ensuring staff remain motived to continue to progress within the department is having clear development pathways, setting realistic expectations from the start as well as providing a supportive environment.

Lifestyle Changes

Life can also change. Priorities can change – the adrenaline of working in an ED can be replaced by a desire for a 9-5 job. Starting or expanding a family can impact on decisions about what job to do and where to live. There can be a desire for travel – to do aid work overseas for a different sense of fulfilment or for the experience of working and living abroad. This has a significant impact on retention, particularly in London. High cost of living and lack of affordable housing was reported as a major factor in the decision to leave urban areas [7]. As nurses look to buy a home, they often find themselves priced out of London with the option of a long commute into work or looking for new opportunities closer to their home. This loss of experienced nurses brings new opportunity for young nurses looking for progression and the experience that London has to offer.

FUTURE DIRECTIONS

The concept of occupational stress and burnout in nursing is not new. However, more needs to be done to ensure the well-being of staff in the NHS, in order to retain skilled and experienced nurses. Current government policy has recognised that this is a significant workforce issue for the NHS and there is a focus on improving retention and workforce development. Retention strategies include addressing remuneration, progression for careers and the immediate work environment [7].

It is important to:

- Provide a supportive workplace culture
- Provide developmental and training opportunities
- Have organisational awareness and action on staff issues
- Support mental well-being

There are a number of priority areas identified in the exit interviews which would help in decreasing the occupational stress and improve the experiences of the nurses working in these areas.

- Reducing overcrowding and improving flow through EDs.
- End corridor care. This is a practice that is undignified for patients, and a major cause of frustration for the professionals caring for them.
- Improve the patient experience – particularly for elderly and frail population. Crowding and long waits for treatment and admission to hospital beds contribute to a deterioration in care and experience for the patients.
- Rota management is a continuous source of frustration, compounded by staff shortages – improvements in retention will help address this. Additionally, if nurses feel more in control of their rota, whether this is through self-rostering, choice of a pattern or having access to a timely rota to plan ahead. Further work should also be done to address the length of shifts and the impact that has on retention, stress, satisfaction, patient experiences.
- How to effectively debrief in EDs?

These are a few of the issues that have been highlighted as nurses have left emergency nursing. These can be taken forwards which can improve the nursing experience, the provision of care and ultimately retention in emergency nursing.

REFERENCES

1. NHS (2019). The NHS long term plan. https://www.longtermplan.nhs.uk/ (accessed 30 June 2020).
2. NHS Digital (2019). Hospital accident & emergency activity 2018-19: NHS Digital. https://digital.nhs.uk/data-and-information/publications/statistical/hospital-accident--emergency-activity/2018-19 (accessed 30 June 2020).
3. NHS Improvement (2018). Performance of the NHS Provider sector for the quarter ended 30th June 2018 2019. https://improvement.nhs.uk/resources/quarterly-performance-nhs-provider-sector-quarter-1-201819/ (accessed 30 June 2020).
4. Royal College of Nursing (2018). Left to chance: the health and care nursing workforce supply in England. https://www.rcn.org.uk/professional-development/publications/pdf-006682 (accessed 30 June 2020).
5. Beech, J., Bottery, S., Charlesworth, A. et al. (2019). Closing the gap healthcare workforce full report. https://www.kingsfund.org.uk/publications/closing-gap-health-care-workforce (accessed 30 June 2020).
6. The Conservative Party (2020). Our plan: conservative manifesto 2019. https://www.conservatives.com/our-plan (accessed 30 June 2020).
7. Drennan, V.M., Halter, M., Gale, J., and Harris, R. (2016). Retaining nurses in metropolitan areas: insights from senior nurse and human resource managers. *Journal of Nursing Management* 24 (8): 1041–1048.
8. Smith, J., Keating, L., Flowerdew, L. et al. (2017). An emergency medicine research priority setting partnership to establish the top 10 research priorities in emergency medicine. *Emergency Medicine Journal* 34 (7): 454–456.
9. Nursing RCo (2017). National Curricumum and Competency Framework: Royal College of Nursing. https://www.rcn.org.uk/professional-development/publications/pub-005883
10. Gillespie, M. and Melby, V. (2003). Burnout among nursing staff in accident and emergency and acute medicine: a comparative study. *Journal of Clinical Nursing* 12 (6): 842–851.
11. Maslach, C. and Jackson, S. (1982). Burnout in health professionals: a social psychological analysis. In: *Social Psychology of Health and Illness* (eds. G. Sanders and J. Suls), 227–251. Hillsdale, New Jersey: Lawrence Erlbaum.
12. Dominguez-Gomez, E. and Rutledge, D.N. (2009). Prevalence of secondary traumatic stress among emergency nurses. *Journal of Emergency Nursing* 35 (3): 199–204.
13. Flint, A. and Webster, J. (2013). Exit interviews to reduce turnover amongst healthcare professionals (Review). *Cochrane Database of Systematic Reviews* 28 (3): CD006620.

14. Morrison, L.E. and Joy, J.P. (2016). Secondary traumatic stress in the emergency department. *Journal of Advanced Nursing* 72 (11): 2894–2906.

15. Allen, R.C. and Palk, G. (2018). Development of recommendations and guidelines for strengthening resilience in emergency department nurses. *Traumatology* 24 (2): 148–156.

16. Edwards, D. and Burnard, P. (2003). A systematic review of stress and stress management interventions for mental health nurses. *Journal of Advanced Nursing* 42 (2): 169–200.

17. Silvester, S., Allen, H., Withey, C. et al. (1994). *The Provision of Medical Services to Sick Doctors. A Conspiracy of Friendliness?* London: Nuffield Provincial Hospitals Trust https://www.nuffieldtrust.org.uk/research/the-provision-of-medical-services-to-sick-doctors-a-conspiracy-of-friendliness (accessed 30 June 2020).

18. Smith-Coggins, R., Broderick, K., and Marco, C. (2014). Night shifts in emergency medicine: the American board of emergency medicine longitudinal study of emergency physicians. *The Journal of Emergency Medicine* 47 (3): 372–378.

19. National Institute for Health and Care Excellence (2009). Mental wellbeing at work: NICE. https://www.nice.org.uk/guidance/ph22/resources/mental-wellbeing-at-work-pdf-1996233648325 (accessed 30 June 2020).

20. Baxter, S., Goyder, L., Herrmann, K. et al. (2009). *Mental Wellbeing through Productive and Healthy Working Conditions (Promoting Well-Being at Work)*. University of Sheffield.

21. Royal College of Nursing (2019). *Employment Survey 2019*. London: Royal College of Nursing.

22. Elmqvist, C., Fridlund, B., and Ekebergh, M. (2012). Trapped between doing and being: Frist providers experienve of "front-line" work. International Emergency. *Nursing Journal* 20: 113–119.

23. Freudenberger, H.J. (1974). Staff Burn-out. *Journal of Social Issues* 30 (1): 159–165.

24. Mateen, F. and Dorji, C. (2009). Healthcare worker burnout and the mental health imperative. *Lancet* 374: 595–597.

25. Graham, B., Cottey, L., Smith, J.E. et al. (2020). Measuring 'Need for Recovery' as an indicator of staff well-being in the emergency department: a survey study. *Emergency Medicine Journal* 37: 555–561.

26. Murray, E., Krahé, C., and Goodsman, D. (2018). Are medical students in prehospital care at risk of moral injury? *Emergency Medicine Journal* 35 (10): 590–594.

27. Litz, B., Stein, N., Delaney, E. et al. (2009). Moral injury and moral repair in war veterns: a preliminary model and intervention strategy. *Clincal Psychology Review* 29 (8): 695–706.

28. Berg, G.M., Harshbarger, J.L., Ahlers-Schmidt, C.R., and Lippoldt, D. (2016). Exposing compassion fatigue and burnout syndrome in a trauma team. *Journal of Trauma Nursing* 23 (1): 3–10.

29. Campbell, D. (2020). Safety fears as hospitals redeploy nurses to care for patients in corridors. The Guardian. Sect. Society (12 January 2020). https://www.theguardian.com/society/2020/jan/12/safety-fears-hospitals-redeploy-nurses-care-patients-in-corridors (accessed 30 June 2020).

30. Smith, P. (2012). *The Emotional Labour of Nursing Revisited – Can Nurses Still Care? Second edition ed.* Basingstoke, Hampshire: Palgrave Macmillan.

31. Smith, P. and Gray, B. (2001). Emotional labour of nursing revisited: caring and Learning 2000. *Nursing Education in Practice* 1 (1): 42–49.

32. Couper, K. and Perkins, G.D. (2013). Debriefing after resuscitation. *Current Opinion in Critical Care* 19 (3): 188–194.

33. Healy, S. and Tyrell, M. (2013). Importance of debriefing following critical incidents. *Emergency Nurse* 20 (10): 32–37.

34. Person, J., Spiva, L., and Hart, P. (2013). The culture of an emergency department: an ethnographic study. *International Emergency Nursing* 21 (4): 222–227.

35. Wallace, J. (2007). Lemaire. On physician wellbeing – You'll ger by with a little help from your friends. *Social Science and Medicine* 64 (12): 2565–2577.

36. Gifkins, J., Loudoun, R., and Johnston, A. (2017). Coping strategies and social support needs of experienced and inexperienced nurses performing shiftwork. *Journal of Advanced Nursing* 73 (12): 3079–3089.

37. Stimpfel, A.W., Sloane, D.M., and Aiken, L.H. (2012). The longer the shifts for hospital nurses, the higher the levels of burnout and patient dissatisfaction. *Health Affairs* 31 (11): 2501–2509.

CHAPTER 8

How Do We Protect Our Healthcare Workers from the Occupational Hazard that Nobody Talks About?

Matthew Walton

National Health Service, London, UK

I became a doctor to save lives. What I did not realise was the closer I was to saving lives, the closer I would be to seeing death. In my final year of medical school, I landed my dream work experience placement with an air ambulance. On the last day, dread set in as we flew towards a horrific trauma. "Possible dead child" came through the radio as we deployed in the helicopter. I had no frame of reference to imagine what we would find.

On landing, we were surrounded by chaos. Flashing blue lights, screaming family members. The child was in traumatic cardiac arrest. I felt lucky that my role was mostly passive. I was free of the pressures of decision-making that lay with the doctor and paramedic. I was in awe of their situational awareness, technical expertise and calm leadership in crisis. To this day, their performance on scene remains one of the most inspiring things I have ever seen. Unfortunately, they were unable to save the child's life. The injuries were too severe.

The scene was disturbing. Images of the child formed permanent memories in my brain. It was a lot to take in. My adrenaline surged, but I still functioned. I was not outwardly upset at the time. Nevertheless, I knew it had affected me on some level. Once we had delivered the child to hospital, a nurse sat me down and told me that it was OK to cry, if I wanted to. Despite the unimaginable tragedy that had just occurred, I did not want or need to.

Back at base, we sat around mugs of tea and debriefed the incident. This helped me to piece together the timeline of what had happened and understand its clinical aspects. We acknowledged the gravity of the case and its potential to be traumatic. I knew this could have life-changing consequences for me. A general practitioner I once met had changed their career after a similar event. But this was my dream job. I wanted to save lives, but could I cope with the reality of witnessing trauma every day, let alone one day becoming the doctor in charge? The doctor I shadowed seemed unfazed and untouchable. Perhaps I was not cut out for this work and my career was over before it had begun?

What worried me most was that I had never been exposed to an event like this before. As a junior medic, I had no track record to assure me that I would come out the other side safely, without developing mental illness. I had met people with severe post-traumatic stress disorder (*PTSD*), anxiety and depression and it terrified me. Their lives had imploded as they lost the ability to enjoy, to form meaningful relationships, and even to feel love. What if the same happened to me? Was it even possible to protect myself from being harmed by what I had seen? Before I went home that night, I asked the doctor I shadowed what to do next. I wanted to know how to begin processing this event. What he told me next changed my life.

He explained to me that I might experience flashbacks, intrusive thoughts and other upsetting feelings after the event. He knew because he had experienced them himself. If the feelings happened or persisted, I should talk about it, even to him. He gave me his mobile number. Sure enough, the case was on my mind for days and weeks afterwards. One night, I sat alone in my car crying, suffering at the thought of the parents' faces watching their child undergoing cardiopulmonary resuscitation (*CPR*). Small reminders triggered visceral reactions. The case was highly confidential so it could not be talked about in much detail with anyone else who was not there. The doctor and paramedic I had shadowed sent me a follow-up message to check in after a few months. All three of us had similar post-traumatic experiences that diminished over time. However, being psychologically affected after a case was stigmatized [1]. We had suffered in parallel silence.

The doctor reassured me that my experience was normal. My sanity was never in doubt whilst my brain slowly worked through the trauma. The basic education he gave me was profound. It was not taught to us at medical school, despite responder trauma being highly prevalent [2]. A recent study of acute hospital staff showed that 10% screened positively for PTSD symptoms [3]. That is higher than British military personnel after the Iraq and Afghanistan wars [4]. I emailed the Office of National Statistics. The suicide rate of paramedics was double that of the general population [5]. Those who care for us 24/7, even on Christmas day, might one day kill themselves because of their work. I was outraged. How do we protect our healthcare workers from the occupational hazard that nobody talks about?

The first step, of course, is to talk about it. My colleagues and I talked together and then with the world. We set about making our experience into a short film. On TV, we tend to see imagery of stoic 'helicopter heroes' saving the day [6]. The full repertoire of an air ambulance crew is very dark. Mangled bodies, fatal burns, hangings. Nobody wants to see that, or film it. We shield the public and our aspiring responders from the reality of frontline pre-hospital care. Contrast this to the military. We know the full force of the blood, guts, gore and PTSD they face; it is catalogued in war films. Our public perception of this phenomenon in healthcare workers lags behind and the result is a deficit of psychological support for our civilian frontline.

Changing the status quo could have consequences. Even when making our film there were many perceived pitfalls. What if people stopped donating to the Air Ambulance Charity? Organisational reputation is critical to providing patient care. The charity relies on donations to keep flying and it was a risk to show their team failing to save a child and being psychologically harmed. They would be vulnerable to criticism. As an amateur documentary maker, I knew broadcasting a solution risks implying a problem. I would face similar dilemmas in the National Health Service (*NHS*). We convince ourselves the risks outweigh the benefits. However, hesitating to acknowledge our problems limits our ability to learn and progress which is the worst risk of all.

We pushed ahead with filming. I packed my car full of camera gear and set off to meet my colleagues. We reconstructed our traumatic experience and kept our message simple: *these experiences are normal – if you are struggling, you should talk*. The finished film was titled 'Resilience – One Team's Trauma' and released online [7]. We were relieved – it instantly helped those who were suffering alone. One student, after witnessing open-heart surgery at a fatal roadside stabbing, said "this film was there for me when I really needed it."

Sharing that simple educational message became our combined aim. High profile medical conferences like *World Extreme Medicine, Trauma Care* and *NHS Education for Scotland Bereavement* welcomed us with open arms. Stephen Fry, the president of MIND mental health charity, tweeted the film. Lifelines put it on their charity homepage. We soon found ourselves on BBC breakfast sharing our story with six million people. I had the great pleasure of working with an experienced producer to create a BBC Inside Out documentary. It communicated the paramedic suicide statistics to the public for the first time. Prince William featured in it speaking about his struggles as an air ambulance pilot. If the future King of England was openly having a hard time being a first responder, we could be pretty sure of one thing – we were not alone.

Raising awareness and de-stigmatising the issue was just the beginning. The question still remains, how could I, or anyone, healthily navigate a whole career of trauma exposure? Focus was on how we could separate the 'weak' from the 'strong' individuals, screening for personality types that could withstand a psychological beating without becoming ill. The military proved that pre-screening did not work [8] and hinted that something bigger than the individual was at play [9]. Professor Neil Greenberg, a military psychiatrist, famously said "resilience is not found within people, but between people" [10]. The space between high performing medical teams is a goldmine of protective factors that we are yet to discover.

But is it actually possible to prevent PTSD? I contacted Dr Petra Skeffington who lives in Australia. She was the only person in the world who ran a proper trial to find out. She delivered pre-trauma education to fire fighters, but it did not make them less likely to get PTSD, at least in the short term [11]. A six-year follow-up is ongoing.

Perhaps the education did not work, or was it working on something else? PTSD is just one small piece of the puzzle. Negative reactions can be conceptualised as a spectrum. They include acute stress reactions, anxiety, depression, burnout, PTSD and compassion fatigue as well as a new concept called Moral Injury.

Moral Injury is a breakthrough term borrowed from the military. The premise of being upset by something that 'transgresses one's moral code' is easily translated into medicine. Symptoms include the guilt and horror of seeing bad things happen to good people or being a helpless witness to poor decisions from leaders in power. Moral Injury can be a normal, non-pathological reaction. Esther Murray's research on air ambulance students [12] was strikingly relatable to me and it became clear that these reactions were commonplace.

What is a 'normal reaction'? We still do not fully understand where to draw the line. There are also positive reactions. Post-traumatic growth describes being changed for the better by trauma. I saw this when I travelled to Melrose in Scotland. I filmed the story of a Tweed Valley Mountain Rescue Team member who had found a body buried in an avalanche as a newly qualified dog handler [13]. He described almost identical reactions to our air ambulance team. He was upset by the experience, but it also inspired him to become a champion for well-being and undertake the role of Wellbeing Officer for Scottish Mountain Rescue. He developed an induction briefing to educate his responders on reactions to trauma and coping strategies. We combined our film with an expertly edited adaptation of his briefing. Our 'resilience briefing' was embedded into the air ambulance student observer induction. It was unlikely it would prevent PTSD. Though, theoretically, it could improve post-traumatic resilience by encouraging adaptive coping [14].

The briefing received positive feedback and it was nominated for the 'Innovation of the Year' award at the Association of Air Ambulances. The design was not the innovation. The innovation was the novel act of delivering education on this topic to students. Like me, they were relieved to finally formalise this part of their training and start developing the tools they needed to cope. The film we made was then included in nationwide air ambulance training that was backed by Prince William and led by Child Bereavement UK with London's Air Ambulance [15]. I received an email from Cambridge University, my old medical school, asking if they could use it to teach their students. The education I received from the doctor I shadowed on my air ambulance placement was *officially* on the syllabus.

How does this apply to the real world of medicine? My ideals were challenged on entry to the NHS as a junior doctor. Well-being was infamously poor, as documented in Adam Kaye's book, 'This is Going to Hurt' [16]. Trusts were soon rolling out 'resilience training' as a tick-box exercise. In doing so they were seen to have addressed the mental health crisis looming in healthcare. I saw the nonsensical nature of this firsthand. Understaffed wards would lose their doctors for an hour to stick pieces of paper on a chart of emotional, physical, psychological and social factors. The facilitator may never have set foot on a ward. Fledgling medics scoffed from Tupperware boxes balanced on one knee. The bleeps around their necks signalled their workload was creeping up unattended. It meant another late finish for the fourth day in a row.

Resilience training was well intentioned but ill-informed and executed. It proved unpopular with frontline staff [17].

My friend working in accident and emergency sent me this text: "I've been thinking about licking a raw chicken to get a sweet 48 hours of respite. And i'm allergic to chicken." I featured it in a resilience presentation. An NHS consultant stood up at the end and asked me what I would advise they do to help their staff. All I could say at the time was, "more doctors, more time off." The systemic issues seemed too great to try and tackle. I read Kevin Teoh's research [18] and gained insights to better understand the influence of organisational factors. Employees stay late, miss lunch, drown in work, suffer bullying and live through inhumane rotas. Without addressing these issues, traditional well-being interventions aimed at the individual are a drop in the ocean [19]. A shift of focus is required, from the individual to the organisation.

One notice in the staff kitchen of an NHS Trust I worked in epitomised the challenges faced by the NHS. This organisation was chronically underfunded [20]. "Staff are no longer being provided with milk," it read. If a cup of tea in England [21] was a stretch too far, staff well-being was dead. What happened next surprised me. A proactive emergency medicine consultant invited me to improve their workforce's well-being. They opened their mind, surveyed their staff and listened to the issues. Radical change followed. They overhauled the rota and created teams who would stick together for months. They even offered a paid hour per week for team bonding. When the 'firm systems' [22] disappeared so did canteen culture and informal pub chats. I saw this reclaimed with a choc-ice on the grass outside of A+E. The next week a new sign appeared: "Milk for staff."

COVID-19 catalysed this change. Issues that had troubled staff for years resolved overnight. Leaders bypassed the usual red tape and focussed on doing what was right in crisis. Staff well-being was catapulted to the top of the agenda. It was now considered an essential part of the public health response. The European Heart Journal called upon myself and colleagues to co-author a paper [19]. The aim was to guide organisations and teams through supporting their staff. It was refreshing to have a blank sheet of paper to work with. We drew on Professor Richard Williams' research [23] to understand the types of stress staff face in crisis. Primary stressors include the obvious trauma, including triage and death. Personal lives are also affected by the secondary stressors of 'living through' the pandemic. We highlighted that practical and tangible interventions are preferred. Providing food, drink and adequate protective equipment is a mental health intervention [19].

The truth is, many of these organisational stressors existed long before the pandemic [19]. Not all organisational factors are modifiable however, even with the deepest internal reflection. We will always face exposure to traumatic events at work. But, what about debriefing, does that help? Critical incident stress debriefing was lambasted by academics as it was thought to worsen PTSD [24]. People have steered clear since, especially forcing an individual to re-live their trauma [25]. Hence, only 12% of resuscitation team leaders are trained on how to debrief [3]. It is hit and miss if you have a senior who will suggest one.

My first cardiac arrest working as 'the doctor' was a blur until the patient's death was confirmed. I asked my senior registrar for a debrief before they disappeared back to their busy duties. We were able to sit down and un-blur the faces of our chaotically formed team. Individuals introduced themselves and we walked through the timeline of events. We asked what went well and what we could do better next time. One junior nurse was upset. I had no idea it was her first time doing CPR. Gathering together to debrief afforded us the time to acknowledge the gravity of the event, to reassure our team that their immediate reactions were normal and it unlocked the ability to follow each other up. Two days later she told me that she cried before coming into work. This is a significant detail she otherwise may have kept to herself.

Debriefing that solely focuses on the traumatic experience of the responder is not recommended by NICE [25]. Importantly, debriefing should be 'performance-focussed'. Research shows that performance-focussed debriefing does not worsen PTSD and responders actually feel more supported afterwards [3]. The value of debriefing may not be in the act itself, but in the rare opportunity it creates for responders to care for one another. Debriefing also improves subsequent performance by 25% [26]. In other words, there is clear evidence advocating this intervention [27].

So why are we not all making time to debrief? I did not understand the barriers at first, until I started working in areas where cardiac arrests happened more frequently. The issues were magnified in the COVID-19 crisis. In the emergency department resuscitation area, I went from breaking the ribs of a dying patient to assessing and treating another in minutes. Even pre-crisis this was the case. The next patient takes priority. Debriefing is pushed aside, delayed and not done. At first glance the problem seems unsolvable. The most motivated resuscitation team leader cannot stagger emergencies to afford time to debrief. The solution is to rota-match teams and carve out paid and protected time at either end of the shift. If this opportunity for responder care is to be systematically implemented, debriefing must become a mutual priority in our national healthcare culture.

How do you change a culture? Post-arrest debriefing does not feature in the Resuscitation Council UK's life support courses. Neither does any substantial information on how to cope with trauma. I teamed up with the air ambulance doctor I shadowed to present this paradox to them in person. Their exemplary sense of organisational responsibility was summed up in their response. "We have a duty of care to our responders." They vowed to update the syllabus. Education in this vessel reaches every corner of healthcare. Life support, or 'how to deal with a cardiac arrest' is the only course taught to every healthcare provider in the UK. This is how you change a culture.

So, what have I learned? Education is everything. We need to acknowledge our problems to solve them. On an individual level, we must equip ourselves with the tools to process our own trauma in a healthy way. It is a skill that develops over time and should be taught on every syllabus. More widely, we must nurture a culture in which we can speak out if we need help and where a focus on our care becomes routine. There is still much we do not know about how to refine our practice. Research is still revealing more about the post-traumatic experience. We do not know how to prevent PTSD and we are yet to see the suicide rate of paramedics improve. But, there is hope. Mental health support for healthcare workers has accelerated, especially in the COVID-19 pandemic. Driven by motivated and educated leaders, we are becoming efficient at putting resources in the right places to have the most impact.

And have I changed? I processed my trauma and I am stronger for it. My career is not over. I still hope to follow in the footsteps of my senior colleagues. I no longer worry if I have occasional flashbacks and nightmares about cases. I am reassured that this is a normal reaction to an abnormal situation. Neither do I worry if I am not affected when others are. I am unashamed to say that I 'enjoyed' treating a roadside stabbing last month. I follow the science but also listen to the questions and the insights coming from the front line. What makes something traumatic for you, but not for me? Can we ever guarantee that we would not succumb to psychological harm at work? When are we most vulnerable? The bigger picture is becoming clearer by the day but I try not to lose sight of the small things.

When working on a ward with a new colleague, one patient became acutely short of breath. Wide-eyed and gasping, the patient watched as we assessed them. We concluded they might have a potentially fatal clot in their lungs. Thankfully, the patient stabilised. We rushed back to complete our ward duties so that we would finish work on time. It was scary though. My new colleague was quiet. I hesitated. I did not know him well and so nearly did not check in on him before we went home. I am so glad I did. His reply and the weeks after affirmed to me that resilience is found between people: "My dad died of a clot in the lung last year, so yeah, that brought back memories for me." Since that moment we became friends and his performance blossomed. I now make the effort to meaningfully ask, one more time than I otherwise would, "no really, how are you?"

There are more ways than one to save lives.

ACKNOWLEDGEMENTS

I would like to thank the extraordinary friends and experts who have been a part of my journey so far. Steve Coates, Andrew McLean, Sheilagh Matheson, Andrew Hartley, Steve Penny, Professor Neil Greenberg, Kevin Teoh, Dr Petra Skeffington, Dr Ronan Fenton, Mark Hannaford, Sarah McLachlan, Laurie Phillipson, Dr Matthew Nelson, Dr Victoria Timms, Professor Richard Williams, Esther Murray, Tony Stone, Dr Mike Christian.

REFERENCES

1. MIND (2016). Blue light programme research summary. https://www.mind.org.uk/media-a/4862/blue-light-programme-research-summary.pdf (accessed 22 October 2020).

2. Mind (2019). 2019 Ambulance staff survey. MIND. https://www.mind.org.uk/media-a/4847/2019-survey-ambulance-service-summary.pdf (accessed 22 October 2020).

3. Spencer, S.A., Nolan, J.P., Osborn, M., and Georgiou, A. (2019). The presence of psychological trauma symptoms in resuscitation providers and an exploration of debriefing practices. *Resuscitation* 142: 175–181.

4. Stevelink, S.A.M., Jones, M., Hull, L. et al. (2018). Mental health outcomes at the end of the British involvement in the Iraq and Afghanistan conflicts: a cohort study. *The British Journal of Psychiatry* 213 (6): 690–697.

5. ONS (2017). Suicide by occupation: England, main data tables – Office for National Statistics. www.ons.gov.uk https://www.ons.gov.uk/peoplepopulationandcommunity/birthsdeathsandmarriages/deaths/datasets/suicidebyoccupationenglandmaindatatables (accessed 22 October 2020).

6. BBC One (2020). Helicopter heroes. BBC. https://www.bbc.co.uk/programmes/b0087g39 (accessed 22 October 2020).

7. Walton, M. (2018). Resilience – one team's trauma. YouTube. https://www.youtube.com/watch?v=DY60ZOWBvDc (accessed 22 October 2020).

8. Rona, R.J., Hooper, R., Jones, M. et al. (2006). Mental health screening in armed forces before the Iraq war and prevention of subsequent psychological morbidity: follow-up study. *BMJ* 333 (7576): 991.

9. Jones, N., Seddon, R., Fear, N.T. et al. (2012). Leadership, cohesion, morale, and the mental health of UK armed forces in Afghanistan. *Psychiatry: Interpersonal and Biological Processes* 75 (1): 49–59.

10. Walton, M. (2018). Processing trauma: resilience may not lie within individuals, but between individuals. The BMJ. https://blogs.bmj.com/bmj/2018/05/15/processing-trauma-resilience-may-not-lie-within-individuals-but-between-individuals/ (accessed 10 February 2020).

11. Skeffington, P.M., Rees, C.S., Mazzucchelli, T.G., and Kane, R.T. (2016). The primary prevention of PTSD in firefighters: preliminary results of an RCT with 12-month follow-up. *PLOS ONE* 11 (7): e0155873.

12. Murray, E., Krahé, C., and Goodsman, D. (2018). Are medical students in prehospital care at risk of moral injury? *Emergency Medicine Journal* 35 (10): 590–594.

13. Walton, M. (2018). Resilience – the avalanche. YouTube. https://www.youtube.com/watch?v=qabCvFwmNyo (accessed 10 February 2020).

14. Bonnano, G.A., Drozdek, B., Wilson, J.P. et al. (2004). The models of traumatic stress. *Trauma Violence Abuse* 2005 6 (3): 195–216. https://doi.org/10.1177/1524838005277438.

15. CBUK (2019). Air ambulance training partnership. Child Bereavement UK. https://www.childbereavementuk.org/air-ambulance-training-partnership (accessed 22 October 2020).

16. Wikipedia Contributors (2019). This is going to hurt. Wikipedia. https://en.wikipedia.org/wiki/This_is_Going_to_Hurt (accessed 30 January 2020).

17. Huntington, G.R. (2019). Resilience training is a slap in the face. *BMJ* 365: l4176.

18. Kinman, G. and Teoh, K. (2018). *What Can Make a Different to the Mental Health of UK Doctors? A Review of the Research Evidence*. London: Society of Occupational Medicine.

19. Walton, M., Murray, E., and Christian, M.D. (2020). Mental health care for medical staff and affiliated healthcare workers during the COVID-19 pandemic. *European Heart Journal: Acute Cardiovascular Care* 9: 241–247.

20. Full Fact Team (2016). Spending on the NHS in England. Full Fact. https://fullfact.org/health/spending-english-nhs/ (accessed 22 October 2020).

21. NHS (2017). Tea is for trouble. https://www.nhs.uk/news/food-and-diet/tea-is-for-trouble/ (accessed 22 October 2020).

22. Rimmer, A. (2019). The firm: does it hold the answers to teamworking and morale? *BMJ* 365: l4105.

23. Williams, R., Bisson, J., and Kemp, V. (2014). Principles for responding to people's psychosocial and mental health needs after disasters. https://www.apothecaries.org/wp-content/uploads/2019/02/OP94.pdf (accessed 31 March 2020).

24. Rose, S.C., Bisson, J., Churchill, R., and Wessely, S. (2002). Psychological debriefing for preventing post traumatic stress disorder (PTSD). *Cochrane Database of Systematic Reviews* (2): CD000560.

25. NICE (2005). For individuals who have experienced a traumatic event, the systematic provision to that individual alone of brief, single-session interventions (often referred to as debriefing) that focus on the traumatic incident should not be routine practice when delivering services. NICE. https://www.nice.org.uk/donotdo/for-individuals-who-have-experienced-a-traumatic-event-the-systematic-provision-to-that-individual-alone-of-brief-singlesession-interventions-often-referred-to-as-debriefing-that-focus-on-the (22 October 2020).

26. Tannenbaum, S.I. and Cerasoli, C.P. (2013). Do team and individual debriefs enhance performance? A meta-analysis. *Human Factors* 55 (1): 231–245.

27. Bhanji, F., Mancini, M.E., Sinz, E. et al. (2010). Part 16: education, implementation, and teams: 2010 American Heart Association Guidelines for Cardiopulmonary Resuscitation and Emergency Cardiovascular Care. *Circulation* 122 (18_suppl_3): S920–S933.

CHAPTER 9

What is peer support? Co-Creating a Programme

Rebecca Connolly[1], Esther Murray[2], Andrea James[3], Liz Harris[4] and Bernice Hancox[4]

[1] Nottingham University Hospitals NHS Trust, Emergency Medicine, Queens Medical Centre, Nottingham, NG7 2UH, UK
[2] Barts and the London School of Medicine and Dentistry, Queen Mary University of London, London, UK
[3] Brabners LLP Law Firm, Manchester, UK
[4] Paramedic and Psychotherapist, Bridgewater, UK

CONTEXT

The College of Paramedics provides legal support for paramedics going through Fitness to Practise (FtP) Proceedings via Brabners Solicitors. To also address the psychological impact of going through this process, a group of passionate and determined paramedics proposed a peer support programme. This chapter describes how the peer support programme was developed by a group of paramedics, the College, staff at Brabners and a health psychologist working in the field of the psychological well-being of allied health professionals. This multidisciplinary team, under the guidance of paramedic and psychotherapist Bernice Hancox, co-created a training programme and terms of reference for the programme which would be freely available to any paramedic who needed it, anywhere in the UK. Paramedics volunteered to be peer supporters and a group of six underwent training in 2019.

INTRODUCTION

The paramedic profession has one of the highest rates of early retirement, work-related stress, anxiety and suicide within any profession [1, 2]. Paramedics have historically been stymied in talking about mental health; pressures of call acuity and a 'stiff upper lip' culture result in a workplace that seemingly disapproves honest and open dialogue, in a form which could help resolve difficult feelings about extremely traumatic incidents and resultant mental health symptoms. Some commentators suggest that around 73% of ambulance personnel feel that their employer is *never* concerned about their welfare following attendance to critical incidents [1].

Between 2011 and 2015 there were 20 paramedic suicide deaths in England, and the risk of suicide in males was 75% higher than the national average [3]; while there is a general paucity of data concerning mental health and psychosocial problems amongst emergency ambulance personnel, attention from the media highlighting increasing suicide rates has prompted further examination of the factors involved in paramedic well-being.

Perhaps unsurprisingly then, research suggests that paramedics have increased risk of post-traumatic stress disorder (*PTSD*) [4]. A recent meta-analysis showed that the pooled current worldwide prevalence of PTSD in rescue workers in general is 10%, however ambulance staff may have higher prevalence of PTSD than their other emergency counterparts of police and firefighters [5] and may be as high as 22% [6]. It has also been suggested that paramedics have higher rates of burnout (described as a triad of high depersonalisation, high emotional exhaustion and low personal accomplishment) [1].

Reasons for this seem to be rooted in the relationship between stress and illness: characteristics within the pre-hospital environment rather than the individual per se lead to stress [2]. Thus, organisational stress factors such as unpredictability of the work, low social support and fatigue [7], underpinned with repeated exposure to suffering and trauma, the cumulative effect of less dramatic incidents: watching someone lose their independence, or have their life transformed by illness or injury [8] leads to a cascade of symptoms presenting as anxiety, guilt, depression and loss of locus of control.

This is articulated well by Rebecca Gilroy, in an opinion piece for The Journal of Paramedic Practice:

> *Paramedics and ambulance crews see incidences [sic] on a daily basis that the average person may only experience once in a lifetime. On top of this, paramedics are also expected to respond to catastrophic events, such as the Grenfell Tower fire or the Manchester Arena bombing, and continue working afterwards.* [9].

So what helps? What techniques are employed by paramedics in the face of copious barriers to mental well-being? Research seems to suggest that talking over incidents with colleagues is helpful [1], a technique mirrored by doctors and nurses working in Trauma Units [10]. This may be partly because peers can understand the unique, disturbing, and challenging situations that are faced by paramedics, but also there appears to be a reluctance to seek formal occupational health support due to fears around confidentiality and perceived implications to career progression [11].

Working under the auspices of the Health and Care Professions Council (HCPC) – the paramedic national Regulatory Body – and local Ambulance Service National Health Service (*NHS*) Trust guidelines, with the background of being employed in a vocation that is concerned with constant high stress situations, trauma and illness requiring significant emotional investment, it is imperative to manage increased risks of developing mental health symptoms. Thus, supportive management of those in whom fitness to practise (*FtP*) is questioned is necessary.

FITNESS TO PRACTISE (FtP)

Protecting the public and justifying the position occupied by paramedics is a key tenet of the HCPC, the body that regulates 15 health and social care professions, stating that paramedics must have the skills, knowledge, character and health to practise their profession safely and effectively, citing five key areas relating to impairment from the Health Professions Order (2001):

- Misconduct
- Lack of competence
- Conviction or caution for a criminal offence
- Physical or mental health
- A determination by another health or social care regulatory or licensing body [12].

FtP investigations have an enormous impact on paramedics, and account for a significant additional stressor underpinning every aspect of their life. Furthermore, concepts such as 'fitness', 'competence' and 'character' are poorly defined [13], leading to additional legal challenges, debate and stress to the registrant, especially given that misconduct accounts for the largest proportion of FtP cases. Partly due to the exceptional and unpredictable nature of paramedicine, together with the impact of practice on paramedic well-being, occupational cultural barriers and increased demand, paramedics receive some of the highest FtP referrals of all health and social care professions [14].

While nurses receive employment, union and legal support [15], historically no such similar support has been offered to paramedics. This has somewhat been ameliorated in more recent times through the creation of the College of Paramedics (*CoPs*) which offers via its membership, access to specialised legal support and representation in FtP hearings (in certain circumstances.)

There is no academic literature available around the impact that FtP processes has on paramedics, however the general medical council (*GMC*) in 2018 conducted an internal review on its process and the impact on its doctors, finding that physicians generally feel 'guilty until proven innocent' with a sense of accusation and blame [16]. It could therefore be argued that similar sentiment is shared by paramedic staff undergoing similar processes. An anonymous blog by a paramedic who was subject to FtP posted by the CoP on their website reported feeling 'devastated', concerned about being able to provide for his family, and 'humiliated' [17].

PEER SUPPORT

Informal peer support occurs naturally in most workplaces and other settings. The term simply refers to the ways in which people who have had similar experiences share these experiences, perhaps with a view to passing on advice about what has worked best for them, or simply to remind their interlocutor that they are 'not alone'. More formal peer support systems are widely used in the realms of healthcare for both mental health issues, physical health issues and addiction [18] and these groups often grow from the work of volunteers, but can also be instigated by the healthcare setting or other organisation. Scully [19], for example reports on a comprehensive peer support programme developed in Australia to support paramedics with the traumatic nature of their work. Evidence suggests that peer support helps those who access it through processes such as those involving social learning theory, like modelling [20] in which peers demonstrate coping mechanisms which have worked for them, and support their peer in developing their own coping mechanisms. In more formal peer support systems, the supporters will have received training on how to listen, how to respond and support appropriately, and what to do when onward referral for more formal support is necessary.

The GMC recognised that facing investigations is uniquely stressful, and as such commissioned the British Medical Association (*BMA*) to provide an independent, confidential emotional support service run by other doctors. This is termed the *doctor support service* and provides the following:

- Six hours of telephone support from the time a complaint is received by the GMC until the matter is concluded (or from the time notification is received from the GMC), taking place during sociable hours, at mutually convenient times agreed between the doctor supporter and the doctor seeking support.
- Face to face support, subject to availability of supporters, on the first day of a hearing and one further day if the hearing runs for more than a day.
- An orientation visit on the morning of the hearing, if required [21].

In order to address the dissonance between the high numbers of paramedic FtP referrals and few support resources, a group of paramedics together with support and funding from the College of Paramedics established a Peer Support network in which help and support would be provided by people who have either gone through Fitness to Practice or have a good knowledge of the process.

Co-Creating the Programme – What Our Peer Support Entails

Six Paramedics were selected and appointed to the voluntary role of peer supporter following written application and informal interviews. The individuals selected represented a cross-section of the profession, operating in different settings with a variety of roles and experience. Desirable characteristics were identified by the psychotherapist and a panel from the College of Paramedic's Mental Health and Wellbeing Steering Group, and discussion took place with each individual regarding ethical dilemmas, motivation and ideas for developing the role and team. The purpose of the team would be to offer low-level psychosocial support to paramedics undergoing the fitness to practice process, with an emphasis on empowerment, while maintaining appropriate boundaries, recognising their limitations and the potential need for onward referral. Support would be offered over the telephone, and consisted of supportive listening using techniques such as paraphrasing, reflecting back what the other speaker had said and being able to respond to the emotional tone of the conversation (see, for example, [22]). The Paramedics would have either a lived experience or good working knowledge of the FtP process and understand the psychosocial difficulties the individual may experience as a result of any investigation. The training was designed to develop self-reflection within the peer supporters an understanding of the setting and maintenance of boundaries, and confidence in both their capabilities and limitations. Reading the available literature and developing a training package, it is clear that more research is required regarding all aspects of peer support in order to provide an evidence base for future programme development. The main source drawn upon for the creation of the programme was work by Creamer et al. [23]. The psychosocial focus of the support available looks to identify potential distress or signs of mental ill health and encourage and empower the individual undergoing FtP to utilise both internal and external sources of support available to them.

In order to ensure a peer support service which could protect both those using it, and those giving support, the Peer Supporters are required to conform to a code of conduct and sign a confidentiality agreement, with the understanding that these documents set out what would be expected of them in the role, and how they would be supported to operate within the remit specified. These documents would be readily available to individuals accessing the service – who would also be provided with information regarding what will be expected of them as a service user; thus encouraging a relationship of mutual respect and understanding from the outset – enabling the individual to make an informed decision, as it is understood that the concept of peer support can be interpreted in different ways. The Peer Supporters would be required to attend Supervision with a qualified Supervisor as it is acknowledged that the process of supporting others in distress can be distressing in itself; it is also considered good practice as self-reflection is further developed and the support provided discussed and scrutinised to ensure it is safe and appropriate. There would also be ongoing training provided on various relevant subjects by different speakers.

Experiences of Becoming Part of the Peer Support Programme – What Motivates Us?

Bernice Hancox – Paramedic and Psychotherapist

I have 15 years' experience of working within NHS Ambulance Services in a variety of roles. Though I have never been the subject of any FtP concerns, I have always found myself acutely aware of the weight of responsibility that holding a professional registration entails – with an associated feeling of vulnerability; these are feelings that have been shared with me regularly by colleagues over many years.

I joined the peer support team within my workplace prior to commencing training as a Psychotherapist, and quickly identified an internal conflict when I discovered the practice of supervision. Psychotherapy training and practice is underpinned by ethics and thus regular attendance at group or individual supervision is considered essential for ethical practice.

I found this lacking in the service being provided in my workplace and not something that was available so at this point I stepped away from offering peer support and opted to offer training sessions to those individuals who would continue to offer the service to other members of staff, educating them on the process of supervision and encouraging them to consider what may be available to them in this regard. As a priority, my concern was for the supporter to be supported themselves by someone appropriately trained to do so.

When I saw the peer support programme advertised by the College of Paramedics I was keen to learn about their vision and upon establishing they considered support for the supporters a priority. As a corollary I took on the role of Coordinator and worked collaboratively with the college to develop the programme, training package, suite of documents, policies and procedures. I was able to draw together my experience of peer support, my understanding of professional registration and my training, skills and approach as a Psychotherapist to create what I deemed to be a safe, robust, boundaried and fit for purpose service for all involved.

As the service is still very much in its infancy, I look forward to seeing it develop, and establish a much needed system of support for individuals undergoing what can often be a lengthy and distressing process.

Rebecca Connolly – Advanced Clinical Practitioner and Advanced Paramedic

I was introduced to the project through my work as an academic and other involvement with the College together with Andrea James' work on defending healthcare professionals undergoing FtP proceedings. I had already informally supported several paramedics through their FtP journey and so the opportunity to create a formal discrete network with Terms of Reference under the auspices of the College against which a small group of peers could provide a large support network was something that was not only desperately needed, but also offered a unique service to paramedics. The disproportionately large number of paramedic referrals to the HCPC (both employer- and self-led) indicates to me an historical orthodoxy punitive approach to paramedic regulation. While regulation in and of itself is of course a necessary component of professional clinical practise, the support offered to paramedics through any FtP concern was and is sorely lacking, especially when mental health can be attributed to so many of the core reasons of alleged FtP concerns. I therefore see the Peer Support Programme as a method by which we can redress this inequality, give paramedics support when required, and improve the FtP process.

As FtP hearings for paramedics remain the greatest percentage undertaken by the HCPC, and as increasingly news and media outlets report on paramedic suicide there still appears to be little research into how and why paramedics navigating extremely emotional, harrowing, and challenging emergency incidents while also coping with the normal vicissitudes of life manage and maintain their own internal sense of self, mental health and place in the world. It is perhaps unsurprising then, that the challenge of supporting paramedics through their vocation is still stymied by a general lack of understanding and perhaps overly transactional management. I feel the Peer Support Programme gives paramedics that psychological headspace, safe from judgement where they can be supported, work through their emotions and feelings, and ultimately allow them to emerge the other side of the FtP process in a stronger mental position.

Esther Murray – Health Psychologist

I first heard about this project via a colleague with whom I was working on another project. He knew I was interested in peer support as an effective method to support psychological well-being at work. There is extensive evidence that peer support brings something unique to both those offering, and those receiving the support. I work with a lot of professional groups, and as an outsider and an allied health professional I can certainly bring my expertise and the benefit of a new perspective on a situation but I cannot claim to have shared the experience or to know and understand the work on the same level as a peer. Most peer to peer conversations are informal, of course, but having formalised systems in an organisation they can help to embed the idea of psychological well-being and the need for day to day support in the organisation's culture. From a pragmatic perspective also, peers are more likely to be working alongside one another and are thus there for opportunistic conversations rather than the more formal support systems which might otherwise be employed. Sharing knowledge among employees about what peer support is encourages them to recognise that 'just listening' is actually an intervention in itself and moves away from the model which suggests that the only good kind of help is expert help.

I was keen to be involved in the peer support programme for paramedics undergoing FtP because of the specific type of threat which this kind of investigation poses to a person's sense of identity, and the ways in which formal and expert systems such as regulatory bodies can disempower their own members at such times.

Liz Harris – Head of Professional Standards, College of Paramedics

Having worked within an Ambulance Service for over 20 years, the majority as a paramedic, I saw the long-anticipated introduction of professional registration for paramedics at the turn of the millennia. Then nearly two decades later, I read with an unfurling disappointment the publication of the People like us? (2017) report. This report revealed that the paramedic profession is the most likely amongst all of the allied health professions (*AHPs*) to find themselves in front of the regulator, with a self-referral rate six times higher than the average for all the 14 AHPs.

The story of those intervening years is worthy of a text in itself, and the factors behind those stark facts are numerous and complex. But for now, I take from that story my reasons for wanting to work towards establishing a peer support network for my colleagues.

The expectations of registration for a young paramedic profession were filled with a sense of achievement and pride. However, the reality for a profession born from within a quasi-military ambulance transportation service was a journey of trepidation for which nobody had a map.

When complaints were made against paramedics, Ambulance Services increasingly started to use the regulator instead of their own internal investigative process. The Ambulance Services would wait to see what the HCPC said before they decided what to do. Ill-equipped and inadequately prepared colleagues with little or no support from their employer were struck off the register by the regulator. The fear was born, stories were told and myths were created surrounding the HCPC, that the HCPC was punitive, that they are out to get you; it is better to self-refer, because it will look better on you rather than coming from your employer. These stories and behaviours became ingrained in ambulance and paramedic culture.

Complaints in healthcare are inescapable and mistakes are inevitable, we are human after all. But the harm to those making the mistakes and those subject to the regulatory processes has gone largely unnoticed throughout the profession's growth into adulthood. From the moment of realisation of a mistake the impact of the act or omission takes its toll on the clinician. Maybe it will be a short-lived period of reflection and learning, but often the impact goes far deeper and the harm, enduring. The psychological effect and threat to an individual's confidence and professional identity can be significant and devastating.

Paramedics provide care for people from birth to death, in unfamiliar and emotionally intense situations, where dealing with mental and physical crisis is the norm. Both personally, and professionally in my role for the College of Paramedics, my overwhelming desire is to support my colleagues, to allow them to achieve their best, in some of the worst, most isolating and unpredictable settings in healthcare, to feel like someone is there for them, should the unthinkable happen.

The peer support programme is a piece of the mosaic of mental well-being mechanisms and support interventions provided by the College of Paramedics to empower individuals to stay well throughout their careers. I am proud to have been part of its inception and very grateful to colleagues who have been instrumental in achieving this.

Andrea James – Solicitor

I'm a lawyer rather than a paramedic and I specialise in defending healthcare professionals facing fitness to practise proceedings before the General Medical Council, Health & Care Professions Council and other regulatory bodies. I felt strongly about the need to establish a peer support scheme for paramedics – and I approached the College about it back in 2016 originally – simply because I encountered so many very sad examples of mental ill-health in my work. There is a category of fitness to practise case based solely on adverse physical or mental health, but in many ways those cases are only the tip of the mental health iceberg. It's incredible how many cases of alleged misconduct or lack of competence in healthcare professionals actually arise from underlying, untreated mental ill-health. I encounter many paramedics who have lived blameless professional lives and then, suddenly, within the space of 6 or 12 months, they're the subject of several patient complaints or they make multiple small errors. Employers (ironically, mostly NHS Trusts) rarely appear to consider why the professional's behaviour has changed and whether support rather than disciplinary action is more appropriate. Then there are many healthcare professionals who have never previously experienced mental ill-health, but the distress of going through the fitness to practise process has a catastrophic effect on their well-being. The impact of fitness to practise proceedings on any professional is profound. Figures revealed by a number of studies speak for themselves: 28 doctors died by suicide whilst going through GMC proceedings between 2005 and 2013. In 2017, it was found that 5/8 of social workers going through HCPC proceedings actively thought about or attempted suicide. Doctors who have recently received a complaint of any kind are 77% more likely to suffer from moderate to severe depression compared to those who have never had a complaint.

Although I can perhaps recognise a mentally unwell person, or certainly a very distressed person, it is not within my skillset to support them (as distinct from perhaps arranging for them to be examined by an independent expert and using that expert's report as defence evidence). I am incredibly grateful to the peer support programme for filling that support gap.

FUTURE DIRECTIONS

In the future we would like to be able to evaluate the programme so that we can learn more about what works for paramedics using peer support systems, especially about Fitness to Practice in the UK. This should enable us to grow and improve the service and hopefully reduce the very intense distress which some paramedics experience when undergoing this process.

REFERENCES

1. Alexander, D.A. and Klein, S. (2001, 2018). Ambulance personnel and critical incidents: impact of accident and emergency work on mental health and emotional well-being. *British Journal of Psychiatry* 178 (1): 76–81. https://doi.org/10.1192/bjp.178.1.76.

2. Holmes, L., Jones, R., Brightwell, R., and Cohen, L. (2017). Student paramedic anticipation, confidence and fears: do undergraduate courses prepare student paramedics for the mental health challenges of the profession? *Australasian Journal of Paramedicine* 14 (4) https://doi.org/10.33151/ajp.14.4.545.

3. Hird, K., Bell, F., Mars, B. et al. (2019). OP6 an investigation into suicide amongst ambulance service staff. *Emergency Medicine Journal* 36 (1): e3. https://doi.org/10.1136/emermed-2019-999.6.

4. Iranmanesh, S., Tirgari, B., and Bardsiri, H.S. (2013). Post-traumatic stress disorder among paramedic and hospital emergency personnel in south-east Iran. *World Journal of Emergency Medicine* 4 (1): 26–31. https://doi.org/10.5847/wjem.j.issn.1920-8642.2013.01.005.

5. Berger, W., Coutinho, E.S.F., Figueira, I. et al. (2012). Rescuers at risk: a systematic review and meta-regression analysis of the worldwide current prevalence and correlates of PTSD in rescue workers. *Social Psychiatry and Psychiatric Epidemiology* 47 (6): 1001–1011. https://doi.org/10.1007/s00127-011-0408-2.

6. Bennett, P., Williams, Y., Page, N. et al. (2004). Levels of mental health problems among UK emergency ambulance workers. *Emergency Medicine Journal* 21 (2): 235–236. https://doi.org/10.1136/emj.2003.005645.

7. Petrie, K., Milligan-Saville, J., Gayed, A. et al. (2018). Prevalence of PTSD and common mental disorders amongst ambulance personnel: a systematic review and meta-analysis. *Social Psychiatry and Psychiatric Epidemiology* 53 (9): 897–909. https://doi.org/10.1007/s00127-018-1539-5.

8. Johnston, S. (2018). My time as a paramedic and why mental health matters. *Journal of Paramedic Practice* 10 (7): 309. https://doi.org/10.12968/jpar.2018.10.7.309.

9. Gilroy, R. (2018). Mental health: caring for the paramedic workforce. *Journal of Paramedic Practice* 10 (5): 192–193. https://doi.org/10.12968/jpar.2018.10.5.192.

10. Alexander, D.A. and Atcheson, S.F. (1998, 2018). Psychiatric aspects of trauma care: survey of nurses and doctors. *Psychiatric Bulletin* 22 (3): 132–136. https://doi.org/10.1192/pb.22.3.132.

11. Alexander, D.A. (1993). Stress among police body handlers. A long-term follow-up. *The British Journal of Psychiatry: The Journal of Mental Science* 163: 806–808. https://doi.org/10.1192/bjp.163.6.806.

12. HCPC (2014). Standards of conduct, performance and ethics, health professions council documents. http://www.hpc-uk.org/assets/documents/10002367FINALcopy ofSCPEJuly2008.pdf (accessed 17 October 2020).

13. MacLaren, J., Haycock-Stuarta, E., and Jamesb, A.M.L.C. (2016). Understanding pre-registration nursing fitness to practise processes. *Nurse Education Today* 36: 412–418. https://doi.org/10.1016/j.nedt.2015.10.025.

14. Gallagher, A., Zasada, M., Jago, R. et al. (2018). Fitness-to-practise concerns and preventative strategies. *Journal of Paramedic Practice* 10 (4): 163–169. https://doi.org/10.12968/jpar.2018.10.4.163.

15. Munday, D. (2011). Fitness to practise: the journal of the health visitors' association. *Community Practitioner* 84 (8): 44–45. http://ezproxy.nottingham.ac.uk/login?url=https://search.proquest.com/docview/882898349?accountid=8018.

16. Baker-Glenn, E., Marshall, J., and Caplan, R. (2015, 2018). The GMC review of fitness to practise investigations and its impact on doctors. *BJPsych Bulletin* 39 (6): 317. https://doi.org/10.1192/pb.39.6.317.

17. Anonymous (2019). HCPC Hearing: a member's perspective. https://www.collegeofparamedics.co.uk/COP/Blog_Content/HCPC_Hearing__A_member_s_perspective_2019.aspx (accessed 17 October 2020).

18. Graham, J. and Rutherford, K. (2016). *The Power of Peer Support: What we have Learned from the Centre for Social Action Innovation Fund*, 4–5. London: Nesta. https://media.nesta.org.uk/documents/cfsaif_power_of_peer_support.pdf.

19. Scully, P.J. (2011). Taking care of staff: a comprehensive model of support for paramedics and emergency medical dispatchers. *Traumatology* 17 (4): 35–42.

20. Bandura, A. (1977). *Social Learning Theory*. Englewood Cliffs, NJ: Prentice-Hall.

21. BMA (2020). GMC investigation support – doctor support service. https://www.bma.org.uk/advice-and-support/your-wellbeing/wellbeing-support-services/gmc-investigation-support-doctor-support-service (accessed 17 October 2020).

22. Jones, S.M. (2011). Supportive listening. *International Journal of Listening* 25 (1–2): 85–103.

23. Australian Centre for Posttraumatic Mental Health (2011). Development of Guidelines on Peer Support Using the Delphi Methodology. Unpublished report. ACPMH. www.acpmh.unimelb.edu

PART 3

INTERVENTION

CHAPTER 10

The Theatre Wellbeing Project – Evolution From Major Incident to Pandemic

Tony Allnatt

Royal London Hospital, Barts Health NHS Trust, Whitechapel, London, UK

CONTEXT

The latter half of 2017 saw the major incident planning of London's hospitals tested three times in short succession by terrorist attacks. The Westminster Bridge, London Bridge and the Finsbury Park Mosque attacks may not have been on the same scale as previous terrorist action in London, but nevertheless proved a significant stressor for those involved in responding to the incidents. In the operating theatres where I work hundreds of members of staff respond to any major incident call; on the day, they may be part of a team which works on a severely injured patient for many hours – or they may wait in the coffee room for hours before being sent home without any patient contact. The emotional responses to both of these situations are multi layered and complex. On one hand, a highly trained team are dealing with a terribly injured person – a dreadful and stressful situation, but one that they see on a near daily basis, and when they are finished they can leave knowing that they have done their best regardless of the outcome. The other, equally highly trained group, meanwhile, wait; uncertain when, or indeed if, their turn will come to attend to the injured. If unused, this group are left feeling frustrated and annoyed – yet without them the incident would be immediately unmanageable.

The Mental Health and Wellbeing of Healthcare Practitioners: Research and Practice, First Edition.
Edited by Esther Murray and Jo Brown.
© 2021 John Wiley & Sons Ltd. Published 2021 by John Wiley & Sons Ltd.

Underlying both of these groups will be uncertainty – what is actually happening at the scene?, how many casualties will be received?, do they know someone involved?, how long will they be needed for?, who will pick up their children?, how will they get home?; the list goes on.

These questions are familiar to me – I was the anaesthetic coordinator in the operating theatres at a major trauma centre on 7 July 2005, when four bombs were detonated in London – three on tube trains, and one on a bus. The major incident plan was tested to the limit that day. For me, it was a completely unexpected event which not only defined my early anaesthetic career, but also exposed my coping mechanisms to be wholly inadequate which ultimately led to decompensated post-traumatic stress disorder (*PTSD*) four years after the event – relentless anxiety with hyper-vigilance and hyper-arousal, a major depressive episode, and suicidal ideation. I was extremely fortunate to not only be able to keep my job – thanks to a supportive department and highly skilled psychiatrists and psychotherapists – but also to eventually be in a position to think about how best to help those affected by future incidents. I was given the opportunity to share my experiences privately by a fellow consultant anaesthetist, friend and the clinical lead for major incidents at that hospital at the time. She had not only completely updated the major incident policy in the early months of 2017, but actually coordinated the response in theatres on the night of the London Bridge attack. She had previously asked me about staff support after major incidents, but I had not been in a position to help much – I was still very much exploring my own response to 7/7 and trying to rebuild my life and career at that time. However, by the beginning of 2018 things had changed. I had taken the decision to talk openly about my own mental health in order to try to reduce stigma, effect cultural change and acceptance, initially amongst my immediate colleagues and, ultimately, the whole theatre team. Beginning the conversations was not easy – but whenever I did, I was immediately met with support and empathy – and all too often an exchange of experience from whoever I was talking with. I had no idea that so many of my colleagues had, at some time, sought help to manage their anxiety, their depression, their own PTSD, their alcohol or drug intake – the list went on. These conversations led me to conclude that, in fact, it was not the major incidents that were the main problem; it was actually the relentless drip-feed of trauma cases which we see in our theatres which were causing problems. Whether an individual could continue to perform well in the face of daily trauma – sometimes several traumas in the same shift – depended on their pre-existing coping strategies; when these became overwhelmed, burnout, alcoholism, stress and depression – or worse – followed. The department had been a witness to a number of staff suicides in the past decade – yet these were not talked about, and psychological support structures were not obviously available at any time. The importance of self-care, self-compassion, effective restorative behaviours – even acknowledgement that the world class treatment being delivered by the theatre teams daily is an exceptionally challenging environment to work in – was almost completely absent. Unsurprisingly, the top reason recorded for sickness in the department during 2017 was stress or stress-related illness.

DESCRIPTION

When we first began talking about how to make a change there were many questions. How could we make a step change with few resources and no financial support? A colleague had heard about a wellbeing session held for the staff in the emergency department (*ED*), so we decided to meet with their clinical director, who had convened the event. I also spoke to our critical care psychologist for some advice, and the four of us met to try and assimilate our ideas into something which would be accessible, useful and sustainable. A governance structure of some sort would also need to be considered going forward, as would measurement of effect.

To begin with, I was keen to survey the department by way of a confidential, anonymous questionnaire to gauge the current level of psychological distress amongst staff. However, while exploring this option, it became clear that this can be dangerous – for example, what would we do if someone expressed suicidal ideation or some other psychiatric symptoms, triggered by the questions? A safe questionnaire with relevant results would require more time and expertise than we had, so the idea was quietly dismissed.

We all agreed from the start that sessions should be multidisciplinary – nurses, anaesthetists, operating department practitioners (*ODPs*), health care support workers (*HCSWs*) and administrative staff; psychological distress affects all, regardless of role. I was particularly mindful of a comment made by one of the HCSWs after 7/7, who said that he had never taken so many limbs to the mortuary. We also wanted to ensure the sessions would be available to not only the staff in main theatres, but also those in ambulatory care and paediatric and obstetric theatres; this would mean trying to reach a workforce of over 600 people!

The most obvious way to achieve this would be to hold a wellbeing event on one of the monthly education mornings held in theatres; protected teaching for all staff, they are usually used to educate on new equipment, policies and statutory/mandatory training etc. These sessions are normally attended by around 150 people, split into smaller groups for targeted teaching. Bearing in mind that there was nowhere suitable that could hold that number of people as a single group, we decided to divide the morning into three separate sessions in different locations, with people rotating between each room and receiving the teaching over the morning. Each session would last about 45 minutes, with 15 minutes to decompress between sessions. All groups would meet afterwards in the coffee room – later dubbed 'cake therapy' – to complete the event.

The content of each of the three sessions was then discussed. At this first meeting we settled loosely on a general introductory session, a session of experiential exchange and peer support ('Staff Stories') and the third session being something practical to physically encourage stress reduction at work. These sessions would evolve over the next few months.

There were still some potential hurdles. The management in theatres required some gentle persuasion, as did the anaesthetic department – but our timing was extremely favourable, with the beginning of mental health being highlighted in the mainstream media as an important part of society, which meant that in reality, very little resistance to this unique proposal was offered. Once all were in agreement, a date was set for the autumn of 2018. It was at around this time that I contacted a second psychologist from our medical school who had been recommended to me by a colleague as someone who might be interested in staff wellbeing. She was immediately interested, and she joined the team at the next planning meeting. We made some firmer plans – my colleague and I would deliver the introduction to wellbeing session; one psychologist would facilitate a session of experiential exchange and peer support; while the other would hold a workshop on physical methods of relieving physical and psychological stress at work. The sessions were undoubtedly ambitious; the logistics of shepherding 150 people between three local but separate rooms alone was daunting. We also had to find people willing to share something with a group of people, many of whom would be unknown to them. Nevertheless, the date was set, and our planning continued.

We decided to divide the first session into two parts – I would deliver an introduction to wellbeing, then my colleague would introduce a system that provides structure for debriefing teams and individuals after particularly traumatic events. She had already been attempting to secure funding from national and local charitable organisations, something which she would ultimately achieve but would take an additional 18 months of hard work. For my part, I wanted to begin with a light hearted look at wellbeing, followed by some very general ideas for individual restorative behaviours and a formal acknowledgement that the work we perform in theatres can be exceptionally difficult and stressful. I also wanted to explain why I was interested in the subject, how it was very personal to me and why I wanted to make a difference. Additionally I was keen to share my own interpretation of the psychological effect of cumulative trauma, which helped me to understand how it could become so damaging. These were ideas that had developed over time as my own experience accumulated and I had open conversations with my colleagues and asked them about how they dealt with their own traumatic experiences.

The search for people to participate in the 'Staff Stories' sessions initially seemed to be straightforward; we were planning to have three stories per session, and I sent out an email request for volunteers. I made it clear that they could withdraw from the event at any time, up to and including the time immediately beforehand. They would also be interviewed by our psychologist facilitator before to ensure their experiences were appropriate and they would be offered support afterwards as necessary. I approached a handful of people personally, and along with the responders from the email, 10 people were initially keen to be involved. Themes about burnout, workplace-based stress and restorative strategies were posited. However, as time passed, volunteers began to drop out; some were not at work that day or were on night shifts, others understandably felt uncomfortable about sharing their personal stories in front of an audience whose reaction would be uncertain – this whole event was, after all, the first of its kind. The number was quickly reduced to just three; two consultant anaesthetists and a consultant surgeon. Each was willing to relay their experience on their own, and each was coached beforehand as planned.

As the day approached, the event was advertised by email, by announcement during morning briefings, and posters through the department. We were unsure exactly how many people would arrive, so we organised a three colour sticker system whereby people were allocated to a colour group for the morning, and their colour would dictate which session they would attend at what time. An anonymous, confidential feedback questionnaire was designed, for distribution after the third session. The questionnaire was paper-based and very simple, asking each participant to rate each of the sessions on a scale of one to five, with two freehand boxes. The first asked them to identify the most useful part of the day, the second what they would like to see in a future session (if there was another). We also requested that people would make – or fake – cakes or biscuits to share during the final session, 'Cake Therapy', a time to not only chat with colleagues about the event but also a period where help could be offered immediately to anyone who had been affected by the topics covered.

The day itself went largely to plan. Members of staff began assembling at 08:45 hours to receive their group allocation. It soon became clear that the numbers attending were unexpectedly high – in the end, almost 200 in total, pushing the rooms to beyond capacity. After a few teething problems with AV support, the sessions began shortly after 09:00 hours. The anticipation was palpable.

I began the introduction to wellbeing session with a light-hearted look at a wide variety of approaches to wellbeing, finishing with the question which, in my mind, it all boils down to – 'are you OK?' As I began to relay my experience at the major incident of 7/7, all fidgeting and shifting in the audience ceased, and silence descended as I spoke. This was extremely encouraging – my presentation was not in any way slick or polished and I was very nervous – but the message was important and needed to be told, and it seemed people wanted to listen. I continued to describe my path through mental ill health and decompensated PTSD, the various problems I had encountered with finding the right help and how I had almost lost my job as a result; but thanks to the support of my friends, my partner, the anaesthetic department and the skills of the psychiatrists and psychotherapists I was able to be presenting this event to them today. I followed with a brief exploration of the answers to the question I had asked at the beginning – are you OK? – and that waiting for the second answer is often more important than the first, often practised response, finishing with a note about how familiarity can help you recognise when someone is not OK, even if their initial answer is contrary to that. I also raised points about how a one size fits all debrief style was not healthy, and forced early debrief can, in some people in some circumstances actually provoke PTSD. I mentioned psychological resilience as an expression which had started life with a very positive message, about children in Hawaii overcoming abuse and deprivation to become successful individuals ('resilient'), but that it had recently been corrupted by managers in business to blame their staff for mental health problems. It is clear that teaching people how to be resilient in the workplace has limited use – whereas addressing workplace stressors should be the beginning of promoting psychological wellbeing.

My colleague then continued with a video presentation that she had directed as part of her submission for funding for MedTRiM, a formalised system of debriefing after significant incidents. Modified from the well-established TRiM course used by the military, police and fire services, this is aimed specifically at medical incidents in the hospital setting. While recognising that no single approach to debriefing would suit everyone, MedTRiM could be a system which could be incorporated into our wider, fledgeling wellbeing service.

The Staff Stories began by explaining the 'rules' of the session to maintain the psychological safety of all; namely, that confidentiality should be maintained outside the room. Also, that there should be no interruptions once someone had started speaking, and the discussion should be concerning experiential exchange and peer support, not criticism or problem solving. The first speaker was one of our consultant anaesthetists who described her own pathway through burnout and associated problems. This was immensely courageous – it would be true to say that no one really knew how her account would be received – but she delivered her experiences with such honesty and emotional clarity that those privileged to hear her were transfixed. As the story unfolded, people became openly emotional, being comforted by colleagues, as she continued to recount her struggles. Once she had finished, the discussion was opened to the floor, and people relayed their own experiences of work-based stress in expressions of genuine empathy. Several senior consultants were present in the room, who were sufficiently moved by these accounts of staff 'just about managing' to later petition senior managers to make step changes in the way some theatres were staffed. This session had never been intended to be a problem-solving forum, but this moment was a most welcome and unexpected result, and encapsulated the growing feeling that this kind of event was capable of significantly improving working conditions in theatres. The second speaker, another anaesthetic consultant with a role in senior management, also spoke about her struggles with work-life balance and how she had overcome them. When the discussion was opened to the floor however, the comments and questions were not aimed at her story – but more about what she was doing about system problems in theatre. Despite the best efforts of the facilitator, this was a lesson to us – that even if the rules are clear, this type of session is unpredictable. The final speaker, a senior surgical consultant, concentrated on the strategies that he uses daily to cope with the stress he has endured during his career. Three very different approaches, each with important messages which were well received by the room.

The third session explored physical methods to combat stress at work. This was a step change from the other sessions, being physically interactive as techniques to cause mental and physical relaxation were demonstrated and then performed. Although unfamiliar to most participants, these methods were embraced with enthusiasm and people were visibly energised both at the time and long after the morning had been completed. The importance of smiling at co-workers and colleagues, greeting with enthusiasm was explored as a good way to start – and continue – the day.

As the last group sessions concluded, everyone returned to the coffee room where the cakes and other items they had baked or faked beforehand were shared and enjoyed. The atmosphere was incredible, and the immediate feedback that we received was so positive that the months of planning were forgotten. Personally, I was approached and thanked by both close friends and colleagues previously unknown to me. Someone that I had known for 25 years, a consultant surgeon that I had attended medical school with, was the first – his comments humbled me beyond expression. A number of people wanted to tell me about their own struggles, either at work, in life in general, whether with a formal diagnosis of a mental health problem or not. I was stunned to discover that so many people were working with such burdens, but due to the stigma, shame and embarrassment surrounding the topic felt that they could not discuss it with their colleagues. It was these interactions, immediately on the day, which underlined to me the importance of talking about these subjects and the effect it could have.

This was just the beginning. There was an air of excitement and energy in the operating suite that was sufficiently obvious for some surgeons to ask the theatre staff what was going on, what had happened in the morning? Some even expressed that they wished they had attended! The afternoon was undoubtedly uniquely atmospheric. This revealed an unwanted effect too; those staff who had been unable to attend due to emergency work – or even unsanctioned semi-elective cases – were bitterly disappointed that they had missed this innovative event. One of the senior sisters made an impassioned plea for her two theatre teams to be allowed to come to the next event – despite us not even having a definite plan for a second; I immediately committed to her at that time to organise a second event which would be a rerun of the first, as soon as was possible. The questionnaire results reinforced this sentiment absolutely, with all sessions scoring extremely highly, and the only real complaint being that there was inadequate cake!

FUTURE DIRECTIONS

Feedback continued to arrive for months afterwards, either from email, corridor conversations or via third parties. Experiential exchange was most frequently cited as being the most important and useful part of the event, so we decided to run some speciality specific sessions. Each session begins with a summary of the rules, in order to establish a safe space for discussion. Although not strictly 'closed door' sessions, punctual arrival is emphasised as important and interruption is discouraged. The discussion begins with someone having the courage to share an important or painful experience with a group of colleagues. Some attendees will be known to the speaker – others may not. By displaying their own vulnerability, the speaker enables others to safely share their own experiences in a supportive environment. Thus the speaker gains support from their peers, and others have their own experiences and feelings validated. People who are yet to experience a similar event can learn from the accounts being shared, and express empathy too. The anaesthetic trainees now run their own sessions – known as Coffee Club – every fortnight. We have also held sessions for ODPs, senior nurses, and are planning to eventually embed this type of session into the monthly staff education events.

In a subsequent event, we invited our 'improving working lives' coordinator to tell us about some of the National Health Service (*NHS*) discounts and benefits which were available to us, including discounted holidays, salary-sacrifice schemes and free theatre tickets. Her energy and enthusiasm was definitely infectious, and the wide range of things available was genuinely surprising to all of us! One item which really caught the imagination of the participants was early morning exercise classes; however, the ones organised by the Trust were not sufficiently early (or late) to be practical for the staff to be able to attend. Nevertheless, one of our anaesthetic trainees – a yoga enthusiast – volunteered to run a pilot session starting at 07:00 hours in the theatre complex itself – the epitome of accessible wellbeing. We were also alerted to another important health benefit, namely Health MOTs, offered to all staff by the Health and Wellness Centre – these offer staff blood pressure, blood sugar and cholesterol testing, along with lifestyle advice. Once again, problems with accessibility were raised, and it was suggested that these one on one assessments could be held again in the operating theatre suite during working hours.

Shortly after the first event, the department was shocked by two separate developments; one concerning addiction (substance use disorder), the other with a suicide attempt. Both of the people involved were well known and respected, long term members of staff; this served to remind us that these sorts of problems can happen to anyone, and when they do – which they surely will again – they will affect everyone involved. Although completely unconnected, they underlined the need for an organised programme to help staff recognise psychological stress in themselves and others and clarify how and where to get help. This was further reinforced by a high-profile trauma case, which deeply affected those involved due to the particular nature of the patient, the injury, and the outcome. Additionally, this case was widely reported in the press, with several reiterations as the case was examined in the courts and the perpetrator sentenced. With each new report, some of those present suffered flashbacks as their memories of that time were reactivated through the media. This has happened many times in the past, but on this occasion, those affected were more willing to talk to colleagues and thus began to realise they were not alone or unusual for feeling this way. One of them has since spoken at a Staff Stories session at a subsequent Theatre Wellbeing Project event to highlight the issue of repeated reactivation of feelings during the public investigation of such cases. Additionally, clinical managers have become more aware of the pathways for staff to follow when they do show signs of psychological stress and are happier to start the conversation too.

While the vast majority of people will be affected to varying degrees by traumatic cases, not everyone will have the confidence and courage to share their experience in an open forum of peers. This underlines that there can be no single strategy that works for everybody to reduce the long-term burden of work related stress. We are exploring other ways of sharing experiences in a less direct way, for example creative writing and art therapy. We have also revealed a need for people to talk through traumatic cases which they were a part of in the past, a few months or many years ago. Discussing these events after prolonged periods can be very tricky; but frequently the person has been carrying these memories for so long, often having never spoken about them, that any opportunity to speak about them with someone who will just listen sympathetically without judgement results in huge outpourings of emotion and ulti-mately some relief.

There were other themes from the feedback gathered. The issue of having some-where quiet to reflect either alone or in a small group was raised, and it is true to say that the communal tea rooms are organised for functionality – namely tea and coffee making facilities, large TV screens and vending machines. There are no obvious addi-tional spaces which are accessible or could be made accessible for the purpose of quiet reflection, so our options are limited. Nevertheless, we are looking to provide something better than the only option currently available for individual space – the toilets.

Harassment and bullying within the department – both vertically and horizon-tally, some racially motivated – has been raised in the Staff Stories sessions, in feedback, and during personal conversations. The most recent Staff Survey also high-lighted some of these problems. These are all notoriously thorny issues which will be covered in future sessions. Other topics suggested for the future include the effect of ageing on the workforce, and issues specific to women, in particular the menopause and menstruation.

A roadmap for wellbeing in our operating theatres has evolved from the work of the Theatre Wellbeing Project. It naturally begins with self-care, closely followed by self-compassion. Once we know how to look after ourselves effectively, we can begin to take care of each other in the form of active listening and peer support. Education will continue in both large and small groups, hopefully with increasing frequency, which will help us to recognise when self-care is not enough and additional help from either local or external sources will be needed to maintain our psychological health. Finally, ensuring these services are well advertised, confidential and accessible com-pletes the package.

Fourteen months after our first attempt, two further events have been held, each with a similar format. The fourth is being planned and is likely to be similar in nature but with different content. I believe that attitudes have changed and continue to change in our operating theatres as a direct result of the Theatre Wellbeing Project. While the novelty of having wellbeing sessions has mainly dissipated, there remains an enthusiasm to continue with the project in the long term, with initiatives to improve individual mental health, to continue group support, to reduce stigma, to clarify the pathways to internal and external support services, and ultimately to encourage a workplace where wellbeing is a priority and the answer to the question 'are you OK' can be given honestly and is received without judgement or prejudice.

COVID-19 – A POST PANDEMIC UPDATE

The proposed fourth event was postponed shortly after completing the first draft of this chapter, when coronavirus arrived in London and many things changed for my colleagues and I. My clinical commitment increased by 50%, but I was honestly more interested in trying to organise and provide psychological support for my colleagues, while at the same time protecting my own mental health. Honouring my clinical commitments while trying to achieve psychological safety in our operating theatres was the challenge that I undertook during the pandemic.

As the pandemic crept towards the UK, I began to realise how fortunate we had been to have established a wellbeing programme before the outbreak, with some pathways in place which would prove invaluable. However, exactly how to upscale support from once every six to nine months to something accessible and appropriate for large groups was not immediately clear? I sought advice from our adult critical care unit (*ACCU*) psychologist initially, who suggested she and her colleagues could run some 'stress-buster' sessions during the working day, but these proved impractical – even though they were only 10 minutes long and held four times an hour, staff simply did not have time to attend. Within a couple of weeks these were discontinued. Increasing our 'Coffee Club' sessions for anaesthetists proved much more successful, although it soon became clear that they could not remain as protected teaching time during the day as they had been previously. After several iterations trying to balance working patterns and the need for support, they were held three times a week immediately after hours for about 45 minutes for several months. Consultants were also invited, as were trainees from ACCU; unfortunately the latter group finished their shift later than our own trainees, so their attendance was occasional at best. The shared experiences of colleagues undergoing unparalleled personal and professional challenges generated huge amounts of empathy and support. Expressed emotion was sometimes raw and uncontrolled as our coping strategies became overwhelmed, but we maintained a positive narrative by reinforcing that what we were doing was essential, and that all our feelings were normal. At the beginning of lockdown, when anxiety was the main enemy, sessions were extremely well attended, and this level of engagement continued into the peak and well into the tail, when physical exhaustion made rest the priority.

However, it was a serendipitous interaction months before the pandemic that produced a revolutionary wellbeing intervention which changed the course of psychological support for all our theatre staff.

During one of many corridor conversations, it struck me that a lot of colleagues – many of them senior – were feeling vulnerable, anxious and isolated but were not comfortable sharing these feelings with each other or a group. So I began to send out weekly emails to all anaesthetists reflecting on my own experiences and emotions, and highlighting the same from others, while at the same time ensuring that the avenues for support were clear. This proved surprisingly popular, with many people thanking me either in person or by email, and it was one of those grateful people who forwarded the messages onto a manager, and then somehow onto the virtual desktop of our Associate Director for Culture Change, who had been redeployed as the Lead for Wellbeing during the pandemic. Coincidentally, I had spoken to a leadership group she convened about 12 months previously on the topic of wellbeing at work. Thankfully, she made the connection and called me to see how she could help facilitate any support sessions in theatres. This conversation was a huge turning point because not only did she contact the head of clinical psychology (who immediately seconded one of the senior trauma psychologists to help), she asked me what would be the best way to provide support. In a moment of hopeful optimism, I gave her my honest opinion, specifically daily psychologist led sessions in the morning before theatres started – and to my surprise she agreed! The sessions would be open to all theatre staff – nurses, ODPs, HCSWs, anaesthetists and surgeons – and after discussion with the psychologist we decided on holding a variety of sessions to include progressive relaxation, mindfulness and self-compassion, with the aim of providing a moment of calm and focus for the day ahead and to nurture a calmer, kinder, more inclusive work environment. This was in direct contrast to heightened anxiety levels about PPE, redeployment, new working patterns and personal safety which were making even the simplest of theatre cases a major challenge.

As a step change in focus – towards self-care and the needs of individual staff and seemingly away from the usual 'go, go, go' – the move proved overwhelmingly popular with the staff, and was initially well received by the theatre managers. Engagement was very high and provided multifaceted tools for staff to help look after themselves and each other during the day. The move proved prescient, as we began to see new levels of domestic trauma and self-harm arriving for life saving operations in our theatres. This was a side effect of lockdown, driven by alcohol and frustration, revealing serious grievances within families normally tamped by friends and other social support. Equally distressing was the number of seriously injured people surviving to hospital and theatres – probably a reflection once again on alcohol consumption but additionally with quiet roads, emergency response times were decreased meaning that people with injuries which would usually be fatal were arriving alive to us. As distressing cases escalated, we began our mornings with a daily psychological check-in which made a huge difference to morale and team building. The atmosphere in theatres became noticeably calmer, more tolerant – and tolerable. This was summed up very nicely by a comment made during a feedback session by one of our long serving staff members

'I didn't know that there was a different way to start our day. These [self-compassion] sessions have changed the way we work, we think. My head is clear; I can focus better on the job; this is the first time the Trust have ever done anything like this, for me, for us – for the staff. Thank you'. Anon.

Not everyone wanted to sit and engage in mindfulness, self-compassion or relaxation, however, preferring something a bit more physical, so we decided to start sessions of 'self-care yoga' led by one of our anaesthetic trainees initially, who was later joined by one of the consultants as demand swelled. The two sessions would run concurrently and were complimented by an occasional third session where stories could be shared in a small group in a psychologically safe environment, similar to the Staff Stories sessions held in our previous events.

These sessions were held every weekday for eight weeks during which time we received our colleagues returning from redeployment to the ACCU, and were able to welcome them into a supportive environment where they could, if they wished to, share their experiences either in groups or on a one-to-one basis with a psychologist.

While their experiences varied greatly, some themes surrounding their weeks on ACCU became clear. This started with varying amounts of distress on discovering they were to be redeployed – and importantly the manner in which this was delivered, followed by anxiety surrounding the expectation of their role and lack of training (two days), immediate and graphic experience of death and dying, and the largely unexpected impact of holding tablet computers in front of dying patients for their relatives to have a last contact. Despite all this, many of the returning staff talked about a sense of achievement, acquiring new skills and the kindness of the staff welcoming them onto ACCU, and had somehow achieved a positive narrative. For some this outweighed the negative aspects, and they had even achieved post traumatic growth. However, for others, the situation was overwhelming and their return to theatres was accompanied by obvious distress; they were greeted with kindness and understanding. One thing which all those redeployed to ACCU were reassured of, is that without their hard work and dedication there is no way that our hospital would have been able to cope so well with the numbers that we received.

As we began to prepare to get back to 'normal', it was clear that the staff had embraced their morning wellbeing sessions and really valued them – and they wanted them to continue in the long term. Understandably, this caused consternation amongst a tranche of managers who could only see the 'loss' of 30 minutes first thing in the morning as a waste of productivity, and it was decreed that they must stop. Nevertheless, the staff responded firstly with a petition; then a survey was circulated which within five days had a 35% response rate, over 130 responses in total. The results were overwhelmingly in favour of continuing the sessions; despite this, the verdict was that they MUST stop, although only after first reducing them to three times a week for a further four weeks as a compromise from our managers.

It is at this point that I revisited my original point of contact, who I had been updating with all the news and feedback during the previous weeks. She was dismayed at the imminent dissolution of the sessions, and a plan was made to lobby the Trust board with a view to reversing the decision. Simultaneously, the psychologist leading the sessions began measuring the current levels of distress within the department using 'distress thermometers'. With over a third of those completing the exercise registering levels of distress above the treatment threshold, this final part of objective evidence made the case irresistibly strong and a deal was struck with our Chief Executive. We were given permission to continue the sessions twice a week for the next six months, during which time QI projects designed to demonstrate effect on staff and theatre efficiency would be completed and presented to the board, before a decision made for their longer-term continuation. This is one of the greatest examples of compassionate leadership that I have ever come across in the NHS, for which I am extremely grateful.

As a final note, while there were only five questions on the survey, there were also free text boxes, where people poured out their innermost feelings, not just about the provision of support during the pandemic, but also about the lack of support from other major incidents – including after 7 July 2005. It was as if my journey from that day was reaching a close and that I had achieved something that I could never have expected; that is, to provide comfort and support to the department that had sup-ported me during my darkest times, during their darkest time. A long time coming; a career defining moment.

This was encapsulated in a comment from the survey

'This [morning wellness] is very good for me, the mindfulness and relaxation really helps me through the day. It's a shame we didn't have this years ago as the trauma that went on. . . in the old building, from the bombings. It would have been nice to get that out of my mind and thoughts. Maybe talking about it would help. I have been here for over 30 years and this has been a long time coming'. Anon.

CHAPTER 11

RUOK? RU Sure UR OK??

Gail Topping and Ruth Anderson

Scottish Ambulance Service, Scotland, UK

CONTEXT

Mental illness is non-discriminatory – it can affect anyone, irrespective of age, gender, sexual orientation, race or socioeconomic status. However, the prevalence of mental illness does vary amongst these groups. Certain jobs can expose people to a greater risk of developing mental illness. A survey for the Mind Blue Light Programme 2015 [1] revealed that 79.1% of ambulance staff gave a negative rating for organisational support in relation to mental health. It also found that members of the emergency services are more at risk of experiencing a mental health problem than the general population but are less likely to seek support. About 14.5% rated their mental health as poor or very poor compared to only 4% of the general population. It has become increasingly apparent that ambulance staff members are being profoundly impacted by their job and the incidents they may be exposed to during their career. Support for staff suffering from poor mental health should be no different to supporting staff who have suffered a physical health problem or injury.

Gail Topping is a Paramedic who has worked for the Scottish Ambulance Service (*SAS*) for over 20 years. Early in her career, Gail attended a traumatic incident that severely affected her mental health. Six weeks into her probationary period as an Ambulance Technician, Gail responded to an incident that ultimately resulted in the deaths of several young children and their mother – all patients were in cardiac arrest at the scene. Immediately afterwards, Gail was dispatched to an assault without

The Mental Health and Wellbeing of Healthcare Practitioners: Research and Practice, First Edition.
Edited by Esther Murray and Jo Brown.
© 2021 John Wiley & Sons Ltd. Published 2021 by John Wiley & Sons Ltd.

anyone checking whether she was ready to respond to another job after the horrific scenes she had just witnessed. There was no stress break. There was no debrief. There was no follow-up or welfare check. No-one asked, 'Are you okay?'.

During the weeks, months and years that followed, Gail suffered crippling bouts of mental illness, including frequent suicidal ideation, that required several periods of lengthy absence. She became socially withdrawn, difficult to work alongside and disillusioned with the organisation. Although she attended many more traumatic incidents during her career, the level of support offered afterwards was inconsistent and, at times, non-existent.

Thirteen years later, whilst attending to an incident that should have been straightforward, a bystander pulled out a knife and charged directly towards Gail and her crewmate. They were able to run and escaped physically unharmed, but Gail was emotionally traumatised. They were made unavailable in order to provide statements to the police and the team in the ambulance control centre had been completely aware of what had just happened, but no-one contacted them to ask if they were okay. Disheartened, Gail drafted an email to senior managers in the SAS prior to her shift end. She emphasised her disappointment at the lack of support or concern for her welfare. She felt demoralised and undervalued. She felt she was viewed merely as a resource, a call-sign, and not a human being. Gail was due to be nightshift the following night but, after getting ready for work, she broke down sobbing uncontrollably and could not leave the house. She had to call off sick. It had caused flashbacks to the incident that had occurred well over a decade earlier involving the children who died, simply because no-one thought to ask how she was afterwards. These two incidents were many years apart, vastly different in nature, yet the lack of welfare support was staggeringly similar. Gail decided that it was time to try to make a difference for those other staff that we know are living with poor mental health but are too afraid to admit it. It was time to try and eliminate the inconsistencies and encourage all staff to discuss mental health and wellbeing more openly. A meeting was arranged between Gail and Ruth Anderson, a Duty Manager in the ambulance control centre. Ruth suggested that Gail tell her story, certain that the impact would get people talking about the effect their job can have on their mental health. They wanted staff to identify the signs and symptoms of stress, anxiety and depression so that people could recognise when one of their colleagues might be struggling and feel confident enough to ask, 'Are you ok?'

DESCRIPTION

The concept of the 'RUOK?' campaign in the SAS is about reintroducing humanity and compassion for those who work in the caring profession – treating each other with dignity and respect and not being afraid to ask a colleague 'Are you ok?'. Overall, it aims to remove the stigma surrounding mental health in our workplace, normalising conversations on a day to day basis.

The 'RUOK?' campaign started by Gail simply sharing her story with control room colleagues, initially focusing on the welfare of road staff. At this point the campaign did not even have a name – it was simply a discussion between colleagues. However, it quickly became apparent that it was not only road staff who were affected – everyone within an organisation is susceptible to stress and poor mental health. Colleagues were struggling but felt that they had nowhere to turn because no-one seemed to be listening.

Gail and Ruth decided to change the focus from purely patient-facing staff and develop a campaign suitable for everyone. When considering what to call the campaign, they initially considered appealing to the Scottish vernacular and incorporate some 'banter' by calling it 'U awrite?' but felt that this may limit its appeal to only those who are familiar with Scots terminology. So, they thought about calling it 'Are you ok?', but this felt quite formal and a bit too 'corporate'. The advent of modern technology and the almost ubiquitous presence of mobile phones means that most people are familiar with so-called 'text–speak' and use of 'RUOK?' as the title of the campaign would ensure its appeal to younger members of staff without detriment to its attraction to older generations.

'RUOK?' is a suicide prevention charity based in Australia. They encourage people to initiate meaningful conversations with friends and loved ones that could save lives. Ruth contacted them to ask if we could share their message and they granted permission for use of their trademark as well as the material on their website.

Gail and Ruth began to develop their campaign in earnest. They created leaflets to be distributed to all SAS employees as well as a PowerPoint presentation to be delivered face-to-face up and down the country. The presentations were initially offered solely within the Ambulance Control Centres, of which there are three in Scotland. Word started to spread, and they were asked to deliver their presentation as part of Continued Personal Development (CPD) events being held throughout Scotland. It became a grassroots movement within the SAS, developed by staff for staff. It is success is entirely attributable to the support and enthusiasm that was shown by those who have attended and helped to spread the message that some compassion and kindness are needed not just for our service-users, but also for our service-providers. The SAS started to realise the impact this campaign was having as so many people started to talk about it. It was promoted through the SAS's quarterly magazine as well as the Chief Executive's weekly bulletins. Staff members were encouraged to share their own personal experiences through anonymised blogs on the organisation's intranet. The ambulance service has traditionally relied on people sharing stories as part of experiential learning. This campaign recognised that everyone had a story to tell, a voice that needed to be heard. By sharing those experiences, people's stories, barriers can be broken down, conversations can be initiated, and people may start to realise that they are not alone. So far, Gail and Ruth's campaign has had over 500 attendees, mostly from people in their own time on a voluntary basis. Colleagues in the Fire Service, Coastguard and hospital staff have also attended some of the presentations. It has also been delivered to new Technician students as well as the Student Paramedic course at Glasgow Caledonian University.

FUTURE DIRECTIONS

As representatives for the SAS, Gail and Ruth were asked to attend a UK wide project group called Project A, which was tasked with the learning and implementation of best practices across ambulance services UK wide. Part of this project's remit is to determine how to improve the mental health and wellbeing of all ambulance staff. Gail and Ruth spoke about the campaign and now the Association of Ambulance Chief Executives want to adopt the 'RUOK?' campaign in all UK trusts.

They have continued to deliver their presentation up and down Scotland and along the way they have met and been introduced to some key organisations, such as Lifelines Scotland, who are working to remove the stigma of mental health within the emergency services and improve availability of support. The challenges affecting the campaign tend to be the same as every other avenue of the National Health Service (NHS) – time and money. Everyone seems to want things to improve, although there always seems to be budget constraints that limit growth, or the time given to properly embed campaigns such as this.

Gail and Ruth would be keen for mental health awareness to be included in induction training whenever anyone joins the ambulance service. Give them a voice from the outset, preparing them for working in a difficult environment, and teaching them how to recognise when a friend, colleague or they themselves are showing signs of poor mental health. They passionately believe that people need to know that asking for help is not a weakness – it is very much a strength. People who choose to work in this environment are not robots. They are human beings, with feelings, families and the ordinary stresses of everyday life as well as risking potential exposure to traumatising incidents through their field of work. It does not need to be a manager who intervenes initially when someone's mental health has been affected. Managers can be affected too and may also require support. Everyone is capable of looking out for each other, regardless of position or rank. If we do not talk about it, we will never get better at being able to identify when one of us is struggling, start a conversation and potentially signpost them to the help that they need. If mental health continues to be kept in the shadows and stigmatised, we run the risk of losing more people either through staff leaving to pursue alternative careers or, devastatingly, from suicide.

Gail continues to receive treatment for post-traumatic stress disorder whilst serving as a frontline Paramedic in a busy ambulance station. She has been awarded the Queens Ambulance Medal in recognition of her work to reduce the stigma associated with mental health.

Ruth has decided to pursue an operational career in the SAS and aims to commence training later this year, ultimately aiming to become a paramedic.

REFERENCE

1. Mind (2015). Blue light scoping survey – ambulance summary. https://www.mind.org.uk/media-a/4584/blue-light-scoping-survey-ambulance.pdf (accessed 15 September 2020).

CHAPTER 12

The Story and the Storyteller

Rusty

St Emlyns, England, UK

Rusty is a paramedic who was diagnosed with post traumatic stress disorder (PTSD) over a decade after experiencing a traumatic event. He had undergone intense psychotherapy. He has sought to increase the accessibility of, and willingness to undertake treatment by first responders through openly discussing his experiences. This chapter explores this journey as well as the impacts and insights he has gained.

Hi, my name is Rusty, and I have PTSD. For a number of years, I spoke openly about having, surviving and then living with PTSD. Podcasts, social media, blog posts and conferences were used to try to promote the message that not only was it ok to not be ok but also that being not ok is a common occurrence amongst first responders. The goal was to help others and there was an unexpected bonus – the meaning making derived from doing so. At some stages of recovery, this was beneficial, but not always. The response to these efforts to communicate the core message through personal storytelling was deeply impactful for the audience, but at a personal level a price was being paid.

The evolution of response to mental ill health amongst first responders continues. Through the increasingly common occurrence of folk being open about their struggles, more and more responders are gaining insight into their own experiences. This is an improvement, but there have been unintended consequences. Sharing these experiences can mean re-living the challenging aspects of them, even for those of us who have undergone some form of therapy and are no longer severely unwell. What

The Mental Health and Wellbeing of Healthcare Practitioners: Research and Practice, First Edition.
Edited by Esther Murray and Jo Brown.
© 2021 John Wiley & Sons Ltd. Published 2021 by John Wiley & Sons Ltd.

has been less prevalent has been these speakers sharing their experiences of opening up. As each of us responds differently to challenging situations, there is no simple equation to follow. I gained insight into the impact of sharing my story by starting to recognise behaviours re-occurring for this first time since therapy – fatigue, low mood, comfort eating. I had to stop through an expression of self-compassion and now I share my experiences in written form.

This chapter will briefly recap my experience of being unwell and the therapy that saved my life. It will go on to explore what came afterwards and what future direction this movement of looking after ourselves better might take. The story will start at the crunch point of realisation that there was an issue that could no longer be masked.

Rusty, we have had another complaint about you. This was the beginning of the end.

In our professional lives, there are a number of phrases we do not wish to hear directed toward us. In this case, the use of the word 'another' had significance. Spend enough time as a first responder, attending other peoples' emergencies and receiving a complaint is somewhat inevitable. The person or people involved are not having a good day and it remains all too easy to be perceived as not acting as expected. This was not that. This was another complaint from colleagues.

Moving to a new house and divorcing are often described in popular culture as being two of the biggest stressors in life. Having copious experience of one and none of the other, it is difficult to pass full judgement, but what I do find a significant stressor is being perceived as being unprofessional. In a twitter thread a number of years ago, the question was posed: what defines a good paramedic? My answer to that question was a paramedic that other paramedics are pleased to see arriving at big jobs. I stand by that definition, aspired to be that paramedic, but failed to live up to it. My professional performance was being affected by stress, and my reputation was poor. I was affected by low mood, loss of self-confidence and a very short fuse. Anger, and even rage, was never far away.

I had developed a chronic response to stress. This was not the normal acute stress response of a few days or even weeks of being affected after an incident. This was a full blown pathological response that comes with a recognisable label: PTSD. As medical conditions go, it does rather do what it says on the tin – a disordered response to stress. Not returning to normal after a challenging event. PTSD is commonly associated with experiencing a single significantly abnormal big event – a terrorist attack's effect on first responders for example. This was not my case. In my case, there was a gradual erosion of mental health through multiple exposures to less headline-capturing but nevertheless abnormal experiences. 'Normal' is not resuscitation, it is not the witnessing of death, it is not the witnessing of the most vulnerable in our society sick or injured and is certainly not seeing families devastated by loss. Thus, as a first responder, the abnormal becomes common. Common enough in my case to lead to a chronic mental ill health.

This complaint was the straw that broke the camel's back. I had been aware of my own ill health and had even accessed enough medical care to have had the PTSD diagnosed for some time. Over the preceding years, I had employed a dizzying array of coping strategies to keep going to work. Of course, the drive to keep going to work was part of the problem – as professional and personal identities were very tightly entwined. This is more than some work ethic on overdrive, this was a deep-seated need to be 'that' paramedic. Reliable, professional, knowledgeable, calm, you know – the paramedic everyone wants to have on scene.

Exercise, meditation, chocolate, attempting to maximise and optimise family time, and more chocolate were amongst the strategies utilised. Eventually the coping failed, and so did I. I had only one reasonable course of action open to me – go sick. This was a journey in itself. Accepting the 'sick role' requires its own process and in the absence of a fever, a wound or broken bone this was harder. The unreasonable courses of action – attempting to plough-on, or attempt suicide – were thankfully rejected by what little remained of my rational mind.

Self-reporting sickness 'for stress' was a bizarrely emotional experience. The unexpected thing to happen was a worsening of my condition – I had assumed cessation of work would have been a relief. It was not. My GP was amazing and basically said the sickness period would be open ended; but having already referred me to mental health services was limited in what they could offer. This left the very pragmatic, action-based paramedic used to proactively taking care of things, in limbo. Perhaps analogous to rescue cardioplegia or blue light syndrome – survivors who worsen as soon as they are rescued – my symptoms of depression deepened. Lethargy was the order of the day, and it took great effort to achieve even menial tasks. This was also the time of greatest risk – those fleeting thoughts of ending it all were arising more often. Serendipitously, therapy was about to start.

There are a number of therapies available to those who suffer with PTSD. In my simple view, they fall into talking therapies (Cognitive Behavioural Therapy (CBT), Eye Movement Desensitisation and Reprocessing (EMDR) for example) and drugs (anti-anxiety and anti-depression medications mostly). The therapy I had been scheduled for was EMDR. This is currently the gold standard of care for PTSD in the United Kingdom. EMDR therapy is led by a professionally qualified therapist and commonly follows three stages - and it did so for me. Stage one is resilience building. Yes, I know, 'resilience' has become one of the most overused words in discussions around staff welfare and mental ill health. Nevertheless, stage one was ensuring I was strong enough to undertake stage two. Stage two is very demanding and commonly PTSD sufferers need support to be strong enough to undertake it. In part due to the numerous coping strategies I had utilised, the resilience building stage was completed relatively quickly. Essentially it was about building an internal psychologically safe space to return to during any maelstrom of emotional challenge during therapy.

This safe place was mostly developed by developing a visualisation – to which you could return at any point. The skills, habits and awareness developed during those hours of meditation, yoga and endurance exercise may not have kept me fully well, but had utility, nevertheless. My response to this progress was sadly a little egotistical, but knowing things were about to get harder was also a source of anxiety. I entered a loop of self-congratulatory narrative followed by dread, followed by a narrative of 'you need to do this, just crack on'. This loop played repeatedly in between sessions as stage one evolved into stage two. In real life this was a period of weeks. It wasn't pleasant; but was a walk in the park compared to what was about to happen.

Stage two of EMDR was horrible. The very experience (s) that made you unwell – time to go back there. Gone was the 'picture yourself in a safe environment' that was a common feature of stage one. The second stage focused on reframing the traumatic experiences with a view to getting past whatever obstacle had prevented the acute stress response from naturally dissipating. In order to do this, the therapy included some element of re-experiencing the original traumatic incident and examining why it presented a block. This was not a single session's undertaking. It took several sessions over several weeks to unpick the underlying psychological components. These sessions were emotionally shattering and indeed it often took a couple of days to recover from them. Recovery took the form of the features of clinical depression: fatigue, lack of motivation, emotional liability and a craving for the sofa and chocolate-based distraction. The sessions were largely weekly. I have heard that some therapists undertake this therapy in a single marathon session. I cannot imagine how that might feel. I barely managed the 90 minutes each week. After some weeks, improvements started to occur: the impact of the sessions became reduced, recovery times shortened, and inter-session well-being increased. Eventually, it was time to undertake the final stage: future modelling and framing of responses.

During the therapy, it became clear that the initial trigger for the development of PTSD had occurred in the first months of working as a first responder. The inability to process these experiences without developing illness arose from an adverse childhood event. This event had left me perceiving myself as permanently inadequate. Similar events to that first trigger event and the resulting emotional challenge had gradually eroded my ability to cope and function. This occurred over a period of 12 years, until the final descent into severe mental ill health and poor performance. That a childhood event had dictated so much of my adult experience was shocking. Awareness of its impact continues to deepen and there is almost no aspect of my personality and life not impacted by this event. Several years on I am still processing this and feel that the time to seek further help in this task is approaching, but I remain not ready. I often find myself contemplating how life might have been without this experience. I feel that this experience was probably an inevitable part of my childhood and if it had not occurred on the day in question, would have happened in a different context on another day. I have also found myself associating most of the negative aspects of my personality to this event. I can be hard work to be around; and having a permanent internal narrative of inadequacy has clearly contributed to this.

In the third stage, the goal is to build post therapy success by reducing the risk of becoming ill again. This is partially facilitated by attempting to re-frame future responses through visualisation techniques. The experience of this stage was mostly very pleasant despite the anxiety felt in approaching modelling responses to future challenges. You could describe this process as rehearsing and then imprinting a normalised response to mental and emotional challenges. Not only was this stage pleasant, two years later it appears to have been quite effective as well.

During stage two an awareness had developed of some of the other first responders who had experienced the same traumatic events that I had – and I felt an immediate and very strong compassionate response towards them. Of course, naturally, thoughts arose about other first responders and their own emotionally traumatic experiences. Contemplating this compassion led me to the strong conviction to attempt to ease the suffering of others.

With time, this compassion manifested into action, and took the form of sharing my personal story. The latter included social media, podcasts, blogs and speaking at conferences as well as a more general openness in daily life when interacting with others. Looking back, it seems that the daily interactions had, and continue to have, the most positive impact upon personal well-being. This openness has also positively impacted my practice in dealing with patients, most especially with those experiencing some form of mental ill health.

After one speaking engagement, I found myself slipping back into some old habits – feeling drawn to the sofa, box sets on TV, gorging on chocolate, reducing exercise, seeking solitude and feeling tired. This lasted a few weeks, and gradually passed. This was the most impactful reaction experienced to various public speaking engagements but was by no means unique. I noted, with the benefit of hindsight, that this impact had been experienced after all such speaking events.

Speaking at events is something most people find stressful, but the reaction to speaking about my illness was more than that. The impact of speaking publicly about my own experience left me incredibly drained and in a low mood. It became apparent that this activity was compromising my well-being, at least in the short term. This became a very challenging time. I had to accept that this course of action that has been selected in order to help others, may not be sustainable. The alternative was a return to mental ill health. After a meditative process of soul searching and acceptance, I have not spoken at a large event in the subsequent years. I remain open and honest about my diagnosis and experience in conversation but no longer do so in so public or large scale a manner. Instead, I have focused on the written word, where I find it easier to stop, and detach if necessary. This experience of difficulty with public speaking had troubling echoes of the realisation that I was not able to perform sufficiently professionally to be an effective first responder. It was possible to see a journey of self-judgment of inadequacy. Fortunately, the third stage of the EMDR is aimed at addressing this very risk – future challenging events and development of strategies to manage the response. Walking away from public speaking was easier as a result.

Unlike the experience of realising that I was not part of the solution but part of the problem in the professional environment, realising that I might not be able to help others by speaking so openly about my illness did not place me into a spiral of depression. On this occasion, the response to the traumatic event of public speaking and sharing followed the more normal sequence of an acute stress reaction. This is very pleasing. For me, this is validation of the therapy that had been undertaken and a source of optimism regarding the future. I am told that such successes are meaningful. I am mostly just grateful I did not become catastrophically unwell again. Perspective is everything.

The experience of having PTSD for over a decade has left its mark. How could it not? Fortunately, the therapy has also left its mark, and I remain well. My sleep remains affected, but the nightmares have ceased, my mood is more constantly positive, and I am able to work clinically again; though I did not return to a role as a first responder.

Life decisions are now judged through the frame of whether the choice will increase or decrease my well-being. Tolerance of decisions that erode well-being is very low. For the first year after completing therapy, improvements in well-being were noted on an almost monthly basis. Change has now slowed but continues. Life is better, I am better. I put this down largely to the impact of the EMDR therapy and will remain forever grateful to my therapist for her work and my family for their support, without which I may not even be living today.

The benefit of this experience has been to learn to be flexible about self-identity. In terms of the PTSD my personal identity was too wrapped up in my professional successes and failures. I fell into the same trap afterwards and became to identified as 'the one with PTSD'. I now have a more nuanced approach to my identity – or at least I believe I do – and seem the better for it. This nuance is driven by two main things – awareness and detachment. Awareness of my mood and state of well-being, and an improved ability to detach from a situation. This is far from easy and requires conscious effort. Unconscious competence may be a lifetime's work; but is a more worthy quest than clinging onto a delusional self-image. I cannot help but reflect on whether there is some form of preparation that can be undertaken in order to help reduce this pattern occurring in others as well. I find myself reaching for the literature and seeking advice from the experts. There is more work to be done to protect our first responders from the abnormal experiences they encounter at work.

When I joined the ambulance service, the average age of my cohort was 35. We now recruit direct from university and our new trainees and paramedics are over ten years younger. I retain a great fear that these young folk are at even greater risk of mental ill health than my generation were. The tempo of work is quicker, the professional demands are higher and the public's expectations of paramedics have been elevated by many drama and real life television shows.

I feel that if we put all our trainees through stage one of EMDR in training and had mandatory annual check-ups with mental health professionals, the burden of ill health, and the suicide rates would improve. The police and military have the 'qui custodiet ipsos custodes' (who guards the guards), I ask – who is caring for the carers?

CHAPTER 13

Death and Disability Meetings at London's Air Ambulance

Working in a Just Culture

Danë Goodsman and Tsz Lun Ernest Wong

Barts and the London School of Medicine and Dentistry, Queen Mary University of London, London, UK

CONTEXT

This chapter will explore the bi-weekly team meetings called *D&D*, from death and disability, used by London's Air Ambulance (*LAA*) – which are based on a 'just culture' philosophy.

The project arose from our shared observations that the meetings offered colleagues much more than just a forum for managing clinical operations – that D&D was not only a central pillar of LAA's clinical governance system but also enabled the team to educate, develop and support well-being[1] of their staff. Our aim in this chapter is to draw out key elements and experiences of the D&D process with a view to understanding its central tenets, contexts and practices – and thereby to deepen the understanding of this type of collective team working.

The study itself was undertaken using an ethnographic, qualitative perspective. Data were collected through field notes from observed D&D meetings and interviews with members of the clinical team.[2]

LAA – The Organisation

LAA is a helicopter emergency medicine service (*HEMS*) founded in 1989 and based at the Royal London Hospital, UK – delivering advanced trauma care and life-saving procedures outside hospital within the Greater London region. London HEMS

The Mental Health and Wellbeing of Healthcare Practitioners: Research and Practice, First Edition.
Edited by Esther Murray and Jo Brown.

(as was) were the first in the UK to carry a senior doctor and paramedic dyad. This system reduced the death rate from severe trauma by 30–43% (when compared to the traditional paramedic-only systems [2]). Wilson et al. [3] describe the pre-hospital phase as; 'a crucial period, when irreversible pathology and secondary injury to neuronal and cardiac tissue can be prevented'. Thus clinical interventions are focused on the sequealae of physiological effects resultant from traumatic insult and undertaken within minutes of the patient's injury – preferably within the first hour, which is referred to as the Golden Hour.[3]

Just Culture – Some Insights

A just culture, as described by Scott-Cawiezell et al. [4] is: 'An environment supportive of open dialogue to facilitate safer practices'. Tucker et al. [5] describe it as a 'supportive work unit in which members believe that they can question existing practices, express concerns or dissent, and admit mistakes without suffering ridicule or punishment'.

Understanding just culture within the context of the LAA is central to understanding how the notion has been utilised in the D&D setting and the impact this has on LAA colleagues. In his 2012 book Sidney Dekker (a leading author on just cultures) [6] states; 'A just culture is a culture of trust, learning and accountability'. From an organisational perspective he notes,

'When something in your organisation succeeds, it is not likely because of one heroic individual. And when something fails, it is not the result of one broken component, or one deficient individual. It takes teamwork, an organisation, a system, to succeed. And it takes teamwork, an organisation, a system, to fail'.

This message includes; people, systems, teams and working practices i.e. all the elements involved the organisation's culture. D&D embraces these elements in a way that provides support, transparency, accountability and agency[4,5]

The notion just culture is not new; the concept was coined in the early 2000s and has caught the imagination widely especially in healthcare. Frankel et al. [9] comment; 'There are excellent examples of institutions applying just culture principles. . . but to date, they have not been comprehensively instituted in health care organisations in a cohesive and interdependent manner'. We note this point and suggest the apparent lack of traction is because just cultures not only require an alignment of values but also appropriate infrastructures in which to work – D&D serves both these purposes.

Just cultures operate in contrast to 'blame cultures' – which generally seek to establish (often individual) responsibility for accidents, error and mistakes. Such understandings then often become the basis of interactions between management, teams and workers. The broader rationale for the just culture ethos is its echo of Dekker's view: 'people are the solution to harness not the problem to control', 'safety is the presence of positives not the absence of negatives', and, 'safety is an ethical responsibility not a bureaucratic accountability' (in Provan [10]). D&D fosters this type of whole group involvement and demonstrates these as the basis of interactions between individuals, teams and the service. Whilst the LAA's D&D's significantly pre-date Dekker's [6] discussions on just culture his notions provides texts to illustrate the empathies and focus they take and, further, reveals the potential organisational reach of D&D. Dekker's statement (ibid); 'Being able to offer an account of our actions is the basis for a decent, open, functioning society', supplies a clear view of the underpinning values, function and purposes of D&D. It revolves around the idea of 'account of action' specifically from the standpoint that the group does not seek to find or apportion blame, but to learn as much as possible from every interaction and case. We note an interesting paradox here, within business literatures importance is placed on aligning values between the workforce, the management and the organisation – suggesting that to have a genuine just culture the whole organisation must operate within the same value parameters. However, D&D functions at a day-to-day action level with the processes and values intrinsically linked to its form and function and is thereby seemingly unaffected by the organisation as a whole.

Notwithstanding alignment not being central to the D&D process, its actual existence or running must be part of internal or external infrastructure. That is to say, without the meetings taking place – through, for example, having the time – the processes around the development of the team, the governance elements and the general learning and welfare support they afford are unlikely to emerge.

The process of D&D appears similar to what is elsewhere described as 'debrief'. Generally debriefs are viewed as having a positive impact. A meta-analysis from Tannenbaum and Cerasoli [11] noted 'teams who engage in debriefs outperform teams that do not. In fact, well conducted debriefs can improve team effectiveness by 25% across a variety of organisations and settings'. Debriefing after critical incidents is shown to help clinicians process their thoughts and emotions from stressful events [12, 13]. It has also been indicated to promote resilience [14] and improve performance [15]. Thus, it is clear to see from the literature that the well-being of colleagues will be centre-staged by employing such post event discussions. D&D also adds the explicit dimension of just culture.

As part of their operational practice the LAA team does have debriefings immediately after each case attended, which serve to offer support for others at the incident and promote interprofessional teamworking.

DESCRIPTION

D&D meetings are twice weekly events, running between one and two hours and facilitated by an experienced LAA doctor or paramedic. A range of people attend including the team's doctors, paramedics and often the LAA's fire crew and the pilots. Also frequently present are doctors, nurses, paramedics, medical students and other interested parties. The meetings are based on discussions of current cases. The bi-weekly, structured case review meeting was introduced into the service in 1996. It appeared the thinking behind this was to foreground openness and transparency in their operating environment.

Order/process:

1. The facilitator invites everyone present introduces themselves and their roles/background.
2. Cases are selected from the file-box. Discussions generally focus on one case in detail and then two to three briefly.
3. The attending clinician(s) give their personal accounts of managing the case. If the patient has had follow up this is also reported.
4. The facilitator then opens the discussion to all. Sometimes the focus is on a specific aspect(s), sometimes general. They encourage everyone present to contribute.
5. In the final stage, key-learning points are identified and documented.[6]

Case discussions start with a description of the incident given by the clinician(s) involved – using both the run-sheet from the files and their memories of the events. These accounts offer full details; including the time LAA was activated, departed, arrived on scene and the mode of transport – and whether there were any difficulties locating and accessing the patient. The clinicians will also describe the scene i.e. on a motorway or in a patient's home etc., and who was there i.e. ambulance crews, police, fire service, distressed family members, members of the public, etc. The level of detail in these aspects is an important part of discussion. The ease or difficulty extricating and transporting patients from the incident to hospital affects the time it takes to arrive and potentially impacts the interval to receiving hospital treatment – which may have bearing on outcomes. Indeed all these factors may affect the choice of pre-hospital interventions. Individuals involved in the broader scene often become part of the purview of the team (families, friends, police, fire crews, etc.) and, alongside the debriefing aspects, their inputs and actions may be part of the discussions and follow-up.

Significantly, at the end of each case the learning points are drawn out, agreed and documented.

D&D is located within a wider LAA system of governance including clinical governance days (*CGD*), 'sign off' days and D&D meetings. CGD are monthly, day-long events open to a wide usually clinical audience. 'Sign off' days are part of the month long induction for new recruits.

D&D Case Reviews

The following are edited interactions from D&D using extracts from field notes – to give a flavour of these interactions. They show not only the range of the discussions but also the openness of the accounts and even in these brief texts it is clear to see the multifactorial elements of pre-hospital medicine.

The first case involved a patient being hit and trapped under a train. (These incidents are called 'one unders' by the London services and LAA attend approximately 40 per year.)

Extract One

Attending doctor (Dr A): There were several ambulance crews on scene and the fire brigade was on scene. Patient was still under the train. . . (description of what appeared to have happened to the patient). . . and I checked that it was safe to go on the track.

Facilitator: Did you get a sense of the patient's physiology? What anatomical things were you considering at this point, and what was your conclusion?

Attending doctor. He was actively bleeding.. . . To me he looked extremely unwell. . . given the history of the patient, his injury and the location; we decided to fly the patient in. At ED (Emergency Department), the CT (Computerized Tomography) scan found that. . . (detailed description of injuries).

Facilitator: (asking other D&D participants) "So the patient was RSI-ed[7], what do you think about RSI-ing him? Is there any downside to intubating someone with head injury?"

Several participants offering their opinion

Facilitator: (asking the clinician) "Why did you think we should intubate him?"

Attending doctor: "It never crossed my mind that we shouldn't tube him. . ..to me the safest thing to do was to RSI." Dr A explains her thought process behind anaesthetising the patient.

Facilitator: Did you know that's what he (the other attending LAA doctor) thought? I found it interesting that you both thought strongly that we should RSI the patient but with completely different reasons. . . I agree with you, I would RSI him. . . What I think interesting is that you made a decision, you weren't aware of what the other person was thinking. . . there were key decision making points where communication could have been useful.

Attending doctor: I admit that we should've taken a minute to step back and talk about what we think so far. . . (at some point) I was trying to call you but you couldn't hear me because it was too noisy.

The candour and depth of detail is well illustrated here especially through the questions and responses in relation to the RSI and demonstrates the familiarity with the level of scrutiny. It is worth noting that in medicine generally an individual's clinical reasoning is not usually shared, let alone as a matter of course (unless something has gone wrong). D&D serves as an opportunity for clinicians to discuss the cases and situations they encountered and hear what others might have done in the same position – potentially towards supporting (or refuting) their clinical actions and also enabling them individually and jointly reflect on their practice.

The reflections on the attending clinician's clinical decisions and decision-making processes are typical of D&D and in some regards the process is adopting the more nuanced understanding of 'reflection on practice' as examined by Elliot [16] where he talks about 'theory derived from practice' (i.e. praxis). He offers this viewpoint as contrast to the more usual position of theoretical knowledge taking primacy over practice-based knowledge. A position advanced by Ryle [17] in terms of the schism between 'knowing how – knowing that'.[8] D&D follows a praxis-based position with shift to learning from experiences and learning as a 'learned group', wherein colleagues acquire and develop understandings with and from each other. For D&D praxis is a conscious and purposeful meld of practice and theory. We hypothesise that this format of group agency supports individual engagement and contributes directly to well-being. Freeborn [18] in a study on satisfaction and psychological well-being among physicians concluded that 'physicians who perceive greater control over the practice environment. . . and who have more support from colleagues, have higher levels of satisfaction and psychological well-being'.

Extract 2

In the second extract, the case is a fall from height and the patient was given a thoracostomy.[9] The patient unexpectedly went into cardiac arrest. We see the dialogue play out between clinician and facilitator – and the response of the facilitator to the issues for the clinician.

Facilitator: What was the reason to anesthetise her?. . . (Facilitator helped to tease out details of the job to help everyone understand what had happened)

Attending doctor: I didn't think she was bleeding but I couldn't quite explain why. I never had someone talking to me then arrested, and I couldn't put my finger on why, I couldn't explain it. It was frustrating

Facilitator: How carefully did you feel the pelvis do you think?

Attending doctor: Probably not to be completely honest. . .

Facilitator: . . . I got that wrong before, I didn't give it [blood], and I regretted it. . . You were right to give blood but it wasn't for the lack of blood that she died

Attending doctor: I didn't expect her to arrest on me. . . on hindsight I would have given bicarb and calcium

Facilitator: Would you do anything else differently? I don't think you should take it in the way as if it would save her. . . It's a horrible feeling. . . (Responding to Dr B who was upset about losing the patient who had previously been talking) Do you think you needed to do anything quicker? There is definitely learning point for all of us going to these arrests. . .

Attending doctor: Everyone else was fairly chilled, but for me, inside was so maxed out. . .. I didn't feel like everyone was at the same bandwidth[10]. . . it was the weirdest. . .'

This case gives some insight into the issues and complexities of diagnosing patients' medical needs from their outward signs and symptoms.

It also reveals the direct emotional impacts involved in managing patients with severe injuries – with the clinician offering a view of their inner turmoil relating to the patient passing away and the added impact of how their personal state appeared to be in contrast to others in the team. Such conversations are common in D&D, and indeed might well come under a psychological debrief umbrella – but the fact that practice and emotion are reviewed in the same group learning setting gives an broader and arguably more realistic context for the individual and the team to consider what happened and what was done. The additional impacts of emotional responses are revealed and teams can review/discuss how they might be recognised and mitigated as, clearly, emotional distress may affect quality of patient care [19] – D&D offers a space for clinicians to discuss and learn and develop from such events.

Some stressors faced by the team are unique to the pre-hospital world, such as managing mass casualties and exposure to seriously injured people at the place where the injury took place. Alongside this there are the physical and environmental factors such as working outside in the rain, the cold, in confined spaces, in the dark and on lengthy difficult extractions. The team also have to deal with aspects related to managing the public and the scene, etc. [20, 21]. And, as noted, these factors together can impact on the clinicians' mental and physical well-being [22, 23]. D&D offers a forum for wider inputs and discussion than simply the attending team's post incident debrief – which appears to aid the positive processing of events.

As we noted earlier, at the end of each case discussion learning points are recorded. D&D is the setting that continuously reviews the operational aspects of service as it is delivered. An interviewee talked about what this offered the process.

'I think here is a kind of third function. . . which is the kind of flagging of governance issues, be it system failings or gaps in service that the team delivered. Those are the internal factors that we are not happy with something that we've done, or things we need to feed back to external bodies about what they've done that we think could be better or different or whatever. And

occasionally things get flagged up in D&D where either we realise that we just don't know something, or we hadn't anticipated something. So kind of demonstrates the gap in our procedures. And it provides a forum to sit and talk about those and try to understand it. And then someone will have the action point of taking it away or learning about it and try to improve that gap'. (LAA paramedic)

Within the mainstream medical context such access to and discussions of equipment and treatments are not generally part of a department's day-to-day remit and from a quality, well-being and governance perspective we see this form of agency supports fully an engaged and responsive team processes.

Experiencing D&D

This next element looks at how working in a just culture is viewed by participants – the following illustrates a lived understanding:

'Everyone learns from it [D&D] and it's an open, honest, and compassionate kind of environment, where they are not picking fault but they are just trying to make next time better. Whereas I think that culture isn't always as well developed in the wider health service. I think people who are being are more prone - certainly, in places I've worked elsewhere - to see that as an adversarial process, a critical process, rather than an educational process. . .' (LAA doctor)

This account opens deeper implications of the team's desire for a just culture. von Thaden et al. [24] quoting Reason [25]: 'Safety culture are made up of cultures that are just; they report, learn, inform and are flexible. . . just culture creates an atmosphere of trust, encouraging and rewarding people for providing essential safety-related information'.

The following is an extract from a doctor, describing the personal understanding of the effects of the D&D process.

'I think it's good because you get the time to look at a case that either you have been involved with directly and discuss it to kind of think about alternative ways to managing things or to confirm that what you did was right. Or to draw on the experience of other people, and analyse your own practice. . . So I think it's quite useful because it draws on the experience of everyone in the room. On the other side of that, when you are listening to other people's cases, it's good to go through in quite a lot of detail because I like that, it's almost like going on the job yourself. If you hear a story of a case unraveling in front of you, when people go through stepwise what they found, what they saw, what they did, you can think in your own mind what you would do, what you would look out and what you would do next, see what they did and compare to your practice. And it's almost like being on the job yourself'. (LAA doctor)

A further advantage of this framework of case-based learning means that participants can also raise any additional topics related to the instance; from pathophysiology, to signs and symptoms of diseases, to making decisions on life-saving procedures – plus the practicalities of pre-hospital medicine including human factors, team management, location and resources, etc.

Needless to say the process requires a high level of trust to be both engendered and maintained throughout. The idea of sharing all you have done is clearly not without risk at a very personal level. In her paper, Laura Delizonna [26] cites Paul Santagata, Head of Industry at Google, who states; 'There's no team without trust', Their study on team performance revealed that their highest-performing teams all had psychological safety as a common theme. The D&D model of discussion exemplifies this standpoint and indeed illustrates how it can be enacted for a group or team. Santagata also notes; 'who is on a team matters less than how the team members interact, structure their work, and view their contributions'. Google outlined five key elements, which closely mirror attributes found in D&D:

1. 'Psychological safety: Can we take risks on this team without feeling insecure or embarrassed?
2. Dependability: Can we count on each other to do high quality work?
3. Structure and clarity: Are goals, roles and execution plans on our team clear?
4. Meaning of work: Are we working on something that is personally important for each of us?
5. Impact of work: Do we fundamentally believe that the work we are doing matters?"

MOVING FORWARD

This chapter has reviewed D&D meetings at LAA and explored what working in a just culture is like for those in this service. We would like to suggest that the D&D meeting form, which 'roots openness and transparency in [the] operating environment', affords trust and agency in a way not often seen within medical settings – creating a method of team professionalisation that both develops the service and supports group and individual well-being.

From a research perspective we would be keen for others to adopt D&D to see if the benefits of the process could be replicated within other disciplines.

NOTES

1. Where 'wellbeing' is taken generally to mean what is good for a person overall [1].
2. Data collection took place between April and July 2019. Queen Mary Ethics of Research Committee granted ethical approval for the study (reference number QMREC2018) and the project had the consent of LAA.

3. 'The golden hour' is the period of time following injury where medical interventions can substantially and positively reverse the physiological sequealae produced by the bodies' reactions to traumatic insult. The interventions themselves are continually advancing as the science, treatments and technologies move forward. LAA is often the leading team in adapting, developing and testing new ideas.

4. Bandura [7] talks of social-cognitive theory; which extends a conception of human agency wherein people have agentic capability enabling them to influence the course of events, and also includes collective agency, which features proxy and collective forms.

5. Rose et al. [8] noted 'the power of agency as the power to change things'.

6. Often this process of cases review contributes to a rewriting of the team's standard operating procedures (*SOPs*).

7. Rapid sequence induction (RSI) is a method of achieving control of the airway using Intravenous induction of anaesthesia, followed by the placement of an endotracheal tube.

8. Ryle [17] *'Philosophers have not done justice to the distinction which is quite familiar to all of us between knowing that something is the case and knowing how to do things. In their theories of knowledge they concentrate on the discovery of truth or facts, and they either ignore the discovery of ways and methods of doing things or else they try to reduce it to the discovery of facts'.*

9. *Thoracostomy* is the insertion of a thin plastic tube into the space between the lungs and the chest wall – used to treat pneumothorax.

10. Bandwidth a commonly used metaphor in the LAA team. It relates to the individual's capacity to process and use information in the moment.

REFERENCES

1. Ransome, B. (2010). Sen and Aristotle on wellbeing. *Australian Journal of Social Issues* 45 (1): 41–52. http://doi.wiley.com/10.1002/j.1839-4655.2010.tb00162.x (accessed 24 August 2020).

2. Roudsari, B.S., Nathens, A.B., Cameron, P. et al. (2007). International comparison of prehospital trauma care systems. *Injury* 38 (9): 993–1000. https://pubmed.ncbi.nlm.nih.gov/17640641 (accessed 9 July 2020).

3. Wilson, M.H., Habig, K., Wright, C. et al. (2015). Pre-hospital emergency medicine. *The Lancet* 386: 2526–2534. http://www.thelancet.com/article/S014067361500985X/fulltext (accessed 9 July 2020).

4. Scott-Cawiezell, J., Vogelsmeier, A., McKenney, C. et al. (2006). Moving from a culture of blame to a culture of safety in the nursing home setting. *Nursing Forum* 41 (3): 133–140. https://pubmed.ncbi.nlm.nih.gov/16879148 (accessed 6 July 2020).

5. Tucker, A.L., Nembhard, I.M., and Edmondson, A.C. (2007). Implementing new practices: an empirical study of organizational learning in hospital intensive care units. *Management Science* 53 (6): 894–907. https://pubsonline.informs.org/doi/abs/10.1287/mnsc.1060.0692 (accessed 9 July 2020).

6. Dekker, S. (2012). *Just Culture: Balancing Safety and Accountability*. CRC Press.

7. Bandura, A. Exercise of human agency through collective efficacy. *Current Directions in Psychological Science* 9: 75–78. https://www.jstor.org/stable/20182630 (accessed 24 August 2020).

8. Rose, T., Shdaimah, C., de Tablan, D., and Sharpe, T.L. (2016). Exploring wellbeing and agency among urban youth through photovoice. *Children and Youth Services Review* 67: 114–122.

9. Frankel, A.S., Leonard, M.W., and Denham, C.R. (2006). Fair and just culture, team behavior, and leadership engagement: the tools to achieve high reliability. *Health Services Research* 41: 1690–1709. https://www.ncbi.nlm.nih.gov/pmc/articles/PMC1955339 (accessed 9 July 2020).

10. Provan, D.J. (2018). Sidney Dekker: the safety anarchist. *Cognition, Technology & Work* 20 (1): 163–164.

11. Tannenbaum, S.I. and Cerasoli, C.P. (2013). Do team and individual debriefs enhance performance? A meta-analysis. *Human Factors* 55 (1): 231–245. https://pubmed.ncbi.nlm.nih.gov/23516804 (accessed 9 July 2020).

12. Cronin, G. and Andrews, S. (2009). After action reviews: a new model for learning. *Emergency Nurse* 17 (3): 32–35. http://www.ncbi.nlm.nih.gov/pubmed/19552332 (accessed 2 June 2019).

13. Hawker, D.M., Durkin, J., and Hawker, D.S.J. (2011). To debrief or not to debrief our heroes: that is the question. *Clinical Psychology & Psychotherapy* 18 (6): 453–463. http://www.ncbi.nlm.nih.gov/pubmed/21171143 (accessed 2 June 2019).

14. Schmidt, M. and Haglund, K. (2017). Debrief in emergency departments to improve compassion fatigue and promote resiliency. *Journal of Trauma Nursing* 24 (5): 317–322. http://www.ncbi.nlm.nih.gov/pubmed/28885522 (accessed 2 June 2019).

15. Corbett, N., Hurko, P., and Vallee, J.T. (2012). Debriefing as a strategic tool for performance improvement. *Journal of Obstetric, Gynecologic, and Neonatal Nursing* 41 (4): 572–579. http://www.ncbi.nlm.nih.gov/pubmed/22548250 (accessed 2 June 2019).

16. Elliott, J. (1991). *Action Research for Educational Change*. Buckingham: Open University Press.

17. Ryle, G. Knowing how and knowing that: the presidential address. *Proceedings of the Aristotelian Society* 46: 1–16. https://www.jstor.org/stable/4544405 (accessed 24 August 2020).

18. Freeborn, D.K. (2001). Satisfaction, commitment, and psychological well-being among HMO physicians. *The Western Journal of Medicine* 174 (1): 13–18. https://www.ncbi.nlm.nih.gov/pmc/articles/PMC1071220 (accessed 24 August 2020).

19. Hooper, C., Craig, J., Janvrin, D.R. et al. (2010). Compassion satisfaction, burnout, and compassion fatigue among emergency nurses compared with nurses in other selected inpatient specialties. *Journal of Emergency Nursing* 36 (5): 420–427. http://www.ncbi.nlm.nih.gov/pubmed/20837210 (accessed 2 June 2019).

20. Boudreaux, E. and Mandry, C. (1996). Sources of stress among emergency medical technicians (part I): what does the research say? *Prehospital and Disaster Medicine* 11 (4):

296–301. https://www.cambridge.org/core/product/identifier/S1049023X00043168/type/journal_article (accessed 1 June 2019).

21. Alexander, D.A. and Klein, S. (2001). Ambulance personnel and critical incidents: impact of accident and emergency work on mental health and emotional well-being. *The British Journal of Psychiatry* 178 (1): 76–81. http://www.ncbi.nlm.nih.gov/pubmed/11136215 (accessed 1 June 2019).

22. Crowe, R.P., Bower, J.K., Cash, R.E. et al. (2018). Association of burnout with workforce-reducing factors among EMS professionals. *Prehospital Emergency Care* 22 (2): 229–236. https://www.tandfonline.com/doi/full/10.1080/10903127.2017.1356411 (accessed 1 June 2019).

23. Baier, N., Roth, K., Felgner, S., and Henschke, C. (2018). Burnout and safety outcomes - a cross-sectional nationwide survey of EMS-workers in Germany. *BMC Emergency Medicine* 18 (1): 24. http://www.ncbi.nlm.nih.gov/pubmed/30126358 (accessed 1 June 2019).

24. Von Thaden, T., Hoppes, M., Li, Y. et al. (2006). The perception of just culture across disciplines in healthcare. *Proceedings of the Human Factors and Ergonomics Society Annual Meeting* 50 (10): 964–968. http://journals.sagepub.com/doi/10.1177/154193120605001035 (accessed 9 July 2020).

25. Reason, J. (1997). *Managing the Risks of Organizational Accidents*. Ashgate.

26. Delizonna, L. (2017). High-performing teams need psychological safety. Here's how to create it. *Harvard Business Review* (8): 1–5. https://hbr.org/2017/08/high-performing-teams-need-psychological-safety-heres-how-to-create-it (accessed 9 July 2020).

Index

The Mental Health and Wellbeing of Healthcare Practitioners: Research and Practice, First Edition.
Edited by Esther Murray and Jo Brown.
© 2021 John Wiley & Sons Ltd. Published 2021 by John Wiley & Sons Ltd.